# Smart Life: Healthy for Life

## Sean Simonds, PT, DPT, CSCS

**2011**

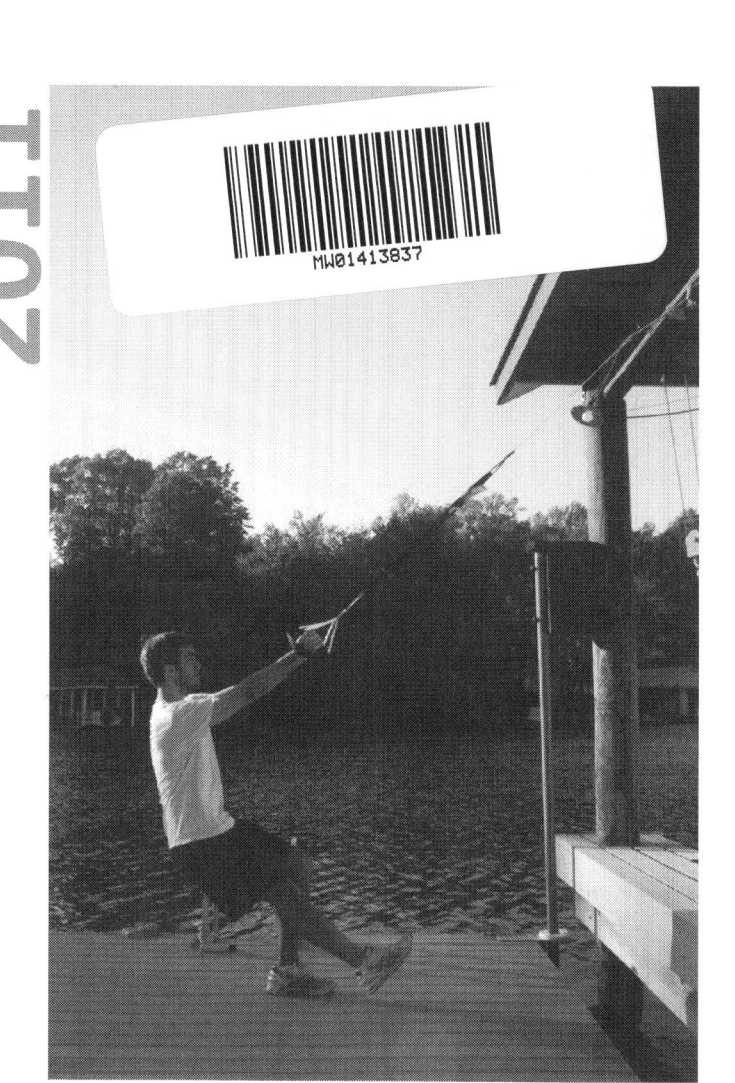

**Smart Life Series**

**www.facebook.com/
SmartLifeSeries**

**smartlife-learninghealth.
blogspot.com/**

**SmartLifeSeries@gmail.com**

**Zazzle.com/smartlife**

Smart Life: Healthy for Life was created to assist you in becoming a healthier and happier person through a series of carefully planned steps. You are given a framework to work within. That being said, you will have plenty of opportunity to individualize it to meet your specific needs. Good luck in this new life adventure you are embarking on!

*To my Ski instructor & fellow boat enthusiast -*

Copyright © 2011 Sean Simonds
All rights reserved.
ISBN: 1468113097

## Dedication

Thank you to my entire, wonderful family. With special thanks to my ever supportive parents and wife.

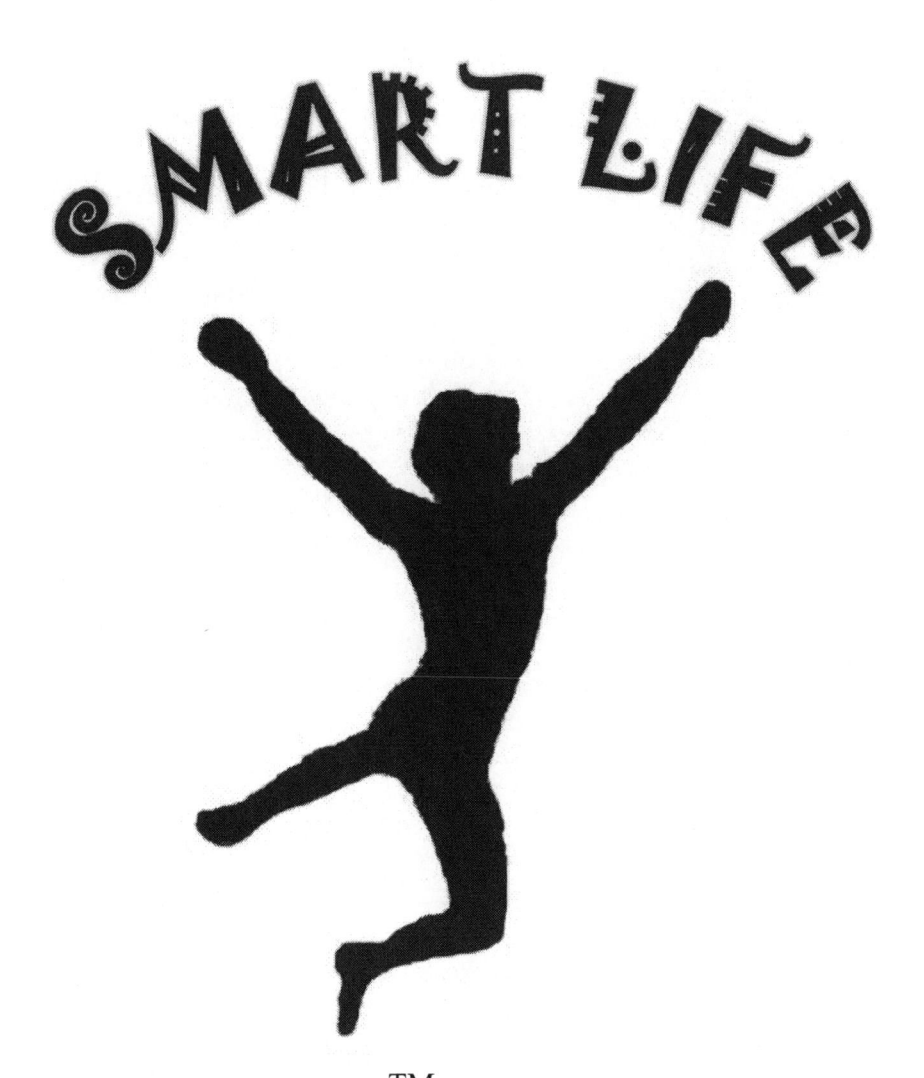

# SMART LIFE

™

## About the Author

**2004-2006:** AFAA certified Personal Trainer
**2007:** B.S. from James Madison University in Kinesiology with a concentration in Exercise Science
**2009:** Earned strength and conditioning specialty (CSCS) from the National Strength and Conditioning Association (NSCA)
**2010:** Doctorate of Physical Therapy from St. Francis University
**2009-2010:** Clinical rotations in in-patient rehabilitation (Gavinana, Italy), pediatric oncology and adult stroke (Morgantown, WV), outpatient sport (Morgantown, WV) and orthopedics (Roanoke, VA).
**2001-2007, 2011-Present**: USSF certified Soccer Referee
**2010-Present**: Physical therapist/clinic manager at two private outpatient clinics in Virginia and PRN work at a rehab facility.

My blog and websites...

www.facebook.com/SmartLifeSeries

http://smartlife-learninghealth.blogspot.com/

Amazon.com: Search for "Sean Simonds"

http://www.lulu.com/spotlight/simondsratgmaildotcom

My other books (currently available on lulu and amazon.com)...

### Smart Life: A Healthier Life at Your Pace
*This book was created to help people change their lives. It supports a life-long change towards healthier behaviors. It is intended for the beginner, but can be used by anyone. The book is set up like a workbook to avoid the monotony of yet another health textbook. It uses simple language to guide the user through a slow, step-by-step process to becoming healthier. It is brief and to the point. It is the first book in the Smart Life Series.*

### Important Italian for the English-Speaking Healthcare Provider
*This book contains useful information/phrases/tips/expressions/and vocabulary for the English-speaker in Italy. It was made for the healthcare provider but contains enough information for anyone to use it to help navigate their way through Italy. The first half of the book contains travel information, tips, and survival Italian. The second half contains information useful to the healthcare provider.*

# Table of Contents

| | |
|---|---|
| Introduction | 7-10 |
| Month 1: Planning Stage | 11-24 |
| Month 2: Motivation | 25-33 |
| Month 3: Diet | 34-60 |
| Month 4: Cardio | 61-76 |
| Month 5: Resistance | 77-87 |
| Month 6: Flexibility | 88-90 |
| Month 7: Planning/Maintenance | 93-95 |
| Month 8: Motivation | 96-100 |
| Month 9: Diet | 101-103 |
| Month 10: Cardio | 104-110 |
| Month 11: Resistance | 111-118 |
| Month 12: Wrapping Up | 119-122 |
| | |
| Index of Exercises | 123-143 |
| Vocabulary | 144 |
| Before and After | 145 |
| Reminders | 146-148 |
| References | 149 |

# **Introduction**

Initial Information

Age: _____        Height: _____        BMI: _____

Weight: _____        Heart Rate: _____        % Body Fat: _____

Blood Pressure: _____        Total Cholesterol: _____

Waist Size: _____        Are you healthy? _____

*Purpose*

    The purpose of this book is simple—to help you make life-altering changes to your health. The entire process will take one year. Before closing the book and scoffing at "one year", give it a chance. The fact is most people who make drastic changes over night are unable to maintain these for any significant amount of time. Eventually, you are back where you started (or worse). This is why fad diets are extremely efficient initially, but fail in the long run. This book will carefully guide you month-by-month through a complete lifestyle change. Progress will be gradual and lasting. It is my hope that, by the end of the year you will be better educated on health and wellness and that you will be a healthier and happier person.

    The program I have developed is presented in a simple manner with a lot of areas for you to record and participate. The plan is supposed to be comprehensive. I will cover diet, exercise, motivation, overall wellness, goals/rewards, etc. I am hoping that this will provide you with all of the tools you need to make these changes and be successful long-term.

    Each chapter will provide you with information, tips and strategies, new goals, and new changes/additions to your life. In order for everything to work, these changes/additions to your life must be kept and carried over from month to month so they become part of your every day life, for the rest of your life. If in one month you walk 20 min/day, you should walk 20 min/day everyday from then on (if this is your goal). Each major topic will be introduced twice. The first time will have a little background and some changes to be made. Then a few months down the road, this same topic will be revisited and you will have the opportunity to expand on these goals and take them to the next level. It is important to point out that you are in control of these goals. I will make suggestions based on things I have done and seen, but ultimately, it will be up to you. Make sure to participate as it will only improve your experience and your chance for success.

    The chart below is showing the major categories (at least in the eyes of the author) contributing to overall health and wellness. Try and come up with a goal for each!

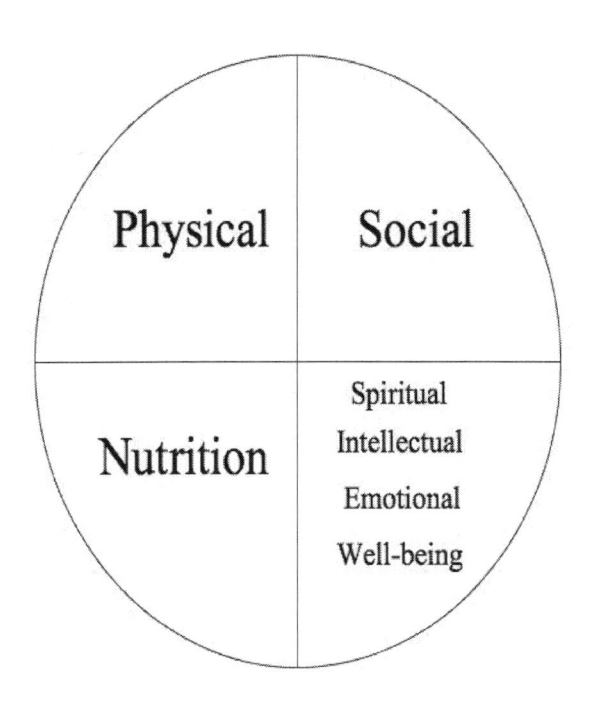

|  |  |
|---|---|
| **Physical** | **Social** |
| **Nutrition** | Spiritual<br>Intellectual<br>Emotional<br>Well-being |

What does your chart look like? What is important to you?

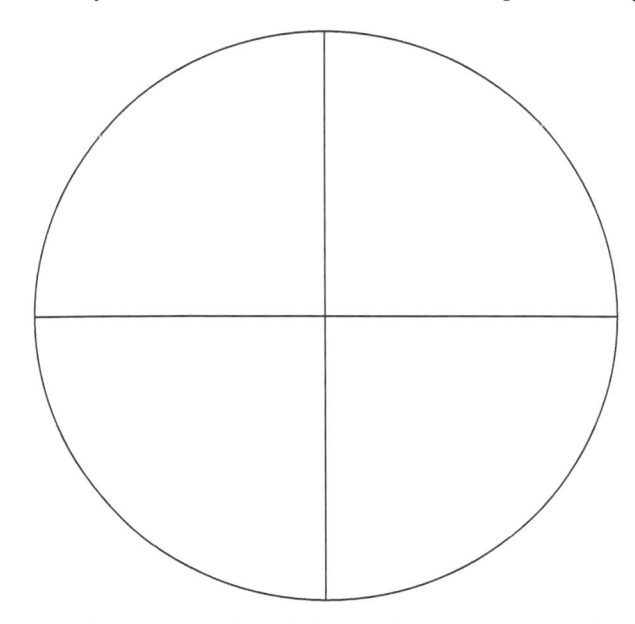

Before we get into things, please complete the goal list below. The idea is to come up with goals you hope to accomplish by the end of this program. I have provided examples of my goals I chose when I started this (yes, I followed the program to make sure it was useful and worked). Feel free to incorporate short and long-term goals. It is the intent of this book to pay attention to all aspects of your health.

---

My sample goal list:
1. Incorporate 30 min of cardio and 30 min of resistance training on 5/7 days/week.
2. Lower my blood cholesterol to 140 (total).
3. Have more energy and feel more relaxed at the end of long days.

---

Your goal list. What you hope to change.
1. _____
2. _____
3. _____
4. _____
5. _____
6. _____
7. _____

8. _____
9. _____
10. _____

**In the space below insert a picture of yourself.**

# Month 1: Planning stage

*Goal: Prepare and organize your life to allow you to begin your lifestyle change. Buy a calendar or a notebook to write everything down in to get started.*

The fact that you have this book means that you are at least contemplating getting started, and maybe you have even begun this journey and are looking for guidance. In either case, I can help.

The first thing you will notice reading this chapter is that there are no recommended changes to your diet, exercise, etc. It is true; this chapter (and much of the next) is all about planning and setting you up for success. These are the stages that never get enough attention and which ultimately lead to people not maintaining their life changes. These stages tend to be skipped. Most people will stand on a scale or get invited to the beach and realize that they have let themselves go. Looking at the extra insulation around their midsection, they think, "Oh shit." Now it is crunch time and they have to lose weight and get looking good fast. No planning or preparation is done and as soon as that beach weekend is over, their lives go right back to normal until the cycle starts all over. This stage is crucial and will allow you to smoothly move through the months ahead with minimal distractions. If you need an extra month, this is the place to take it. You need a solid foundation to set yourself up for success.

In the mean time you should not just sit on the couch and watch hours of re-runs you did not like the first time. As part of this planning month, you need to figure out what you like to do. Try new exercises, foods, sources of motivation (even if it is just one time). Here are just a few suggestions:

*Cardio*: stationary biking, mountain biking, hiking, rock climbing, rowing, kayaking, walking, jogging, running, swimming, zoomba, jazzercise, etc.

*Resistance Training*: free weights, machine weights, suspension bands, rubber bands, body weight, pulley systems, kettle bells, medicine balls, circuit training, etc

*Flexibility*: yoga, pilates, static stretching, dynamic stretching, tai chi

*Diet*: strawberries, melons, whole grains, spinach, nuts, low fat/fat-free options, yogurt, peaches, raspberries, honeydew

*Motivation/Rewards*: food, movies, clothes, intrinsic, concerts, etc.

---

There is a generally accepted framework when dealing with lifestyle change, which we will be following. They are stepping stones that in themselves can act as motivation and goals.

*Pre-contemplation*→ "I do not want to change. I am not ready to change." If you have this book, you're already past this stage!

*Contemplation*→ "I think change is in order…" This is where you are just thinking about changes. No concrete plans, no decisions yet. This is the exact point you are at in this section of the book. Getting ready to prepare, just haven't started.

*Preparation*→ "Time to change, let's get ready." This is a big hurdle and a lot of work for most people. Most of the planning and thinking comes into play here. What are my goals, what do I hope to achieve, what is my budget, what do I need, etc.? This stage is the main focus of the 1st, 2nd, 7th, and 8th month. Four out of the twelve months will be focused on planning. Set the foundation.

*Action*→ "I'm actually doing it!" (Months 3-6, 9-11)

*Maintenance* → "I have changed and I am still doing it!" This is possibly the hardest point to reach. Many people accelerate through the stages and actually get started (action), but then get tired or brush it to the side and go back to preparation. It is an ongoing cycle in most people's lives, always trying to reach maintenance, but never quite getting it. Our goal is to reach this stage and stay here permanently. (Month 12 and beyond)

*Planning Your Exercise*

What do you think you need to do to get started?
1. _____
2. _____
3. _____
4. _____
5. _____

| My answers to the above question were: | |
|---|---|
| 1. Find time | 3. Involve friends |
| 2. Establish a good/supportive environment | 4. Budget my money |
| | 5. Find motivation. |

Time is by far the primary reason for not starting and/or quitting a new routine. The bottom line is that no one has time. Everyone is always strapped for time. You can be a doctor on-call every night, a CEO of a major corporation, a student, or a retiree, no one has time. It is the people who want to change that are able to "find time." Sometimes it can be hidden and you just need to find it, other times it has to be created. If you look at your life and still cannot find even a second of time for physical activity (which many people swear is the case), then you are not looking and/or you do not actually want to make changes. I heard a friend complaining about not being able to find time in their schedule to exercise to which my best friend replied, "Does having a stroke and type II diabetes fit better into your schedule?" A joke, but unhealthy lifestyles, no exercise, and poor diet, have caused a serious health epidemic in this country and the world. Obesity is linked to an enormous list of health problems, increasing healthcare costs for everyone, and premature, <u>preventable</u> death.

The great thing about making calculated changes to your lifestyle is that we are not looking to make enormous time commitments. Our goal is to create a lifestyle that suits you and reduces your health risks.

A very common goal I tell friends and patients who are not used to regular exercise is to start with 15 min/day of walking. It seems simple enough right? Most people struggle to find 15 min/day where they can put everything down and just walk. It is a relatively easy exercise to start with whether you have exercised before or not. I suggest it to you right now. It does not matter if you have a treadmill, a walking path, or you just walk around the outside of your house for 15 min/day, you just have to do it. The great thing about the benefits of physical activity is that they do not have to be done in large chunks. The American College of Sports Medicine and the American Heart Association recommend a total of 30 min/day of moderate physical activity. I am just asking for 15 min of walking. I had a patient recently tell me that she could not fit that into her day. I asked her to record what she did every minute of her day.

6:10am—7: alarm, prepared for work.
7—7:30: drove to work.
8—12: worked
12—1: sat in kitchen with lunch
1—1:10: waited for friend to go to meeting
1:10—3: meeting
3—5: worked at desk
5—5:45: drove home
5:45—7: got changed, made dinner, ate dinner
7—8: paperwork
8—10: TV
Bed

This is a typical day for most people working an 8—5 or 9—5 job. I found at least 6 time slots where a minimum of 5 minutes of walking could have gone. She could set her alarm 5 minutes early and do a quick walk before her morning shower. 5+ minutes could have been done at lunch and waiting for her friend after lunch. After getting changed and before dinner there are easily 5 minutes. Finally, 2 hours of TV time can be used much more productively. At the very least she could stand up and do a lap around her house during some of the commercial time. I suggested these simple adjustments to her schedule and she now walks 20-30 min/day.

### Time you didn't know existed

1. Most people sit while talking on the phone. Stand up and walk around.
2. People sit at their desk at work all day. Rather than checking your email, walk around for a few minutes as your break.
3. Another surprising time is when you are brushing your teeth. Instead of sitting in front of a mirror, wander around the house for the entire time it takes to brush your teeth.
4. Take the stairs instead of the elevator/escalator.

> You do not need to block one and two hour portions of your day off for exercise, especially when you are just getting started! 5 minutes here and there is a great way to start.

Once getting 15 minutes of walking in has become easy, try introducing and extra 5 minutes of something else (stretching, weights, etc.). You do not have to get sweaty and worn out for physical activity to be beneficial.

What are some times in your day you can sneak 5 min in? Do not make excuses, make the time.

1. _____
2. _____
3. _____


*Creating a Supportive Environment*

Environments are tricky. Depending on where and who you live with, you can be in very different situations. The goal here will be making the most of your environment.

If it is just you and your spouse, there are a number of things you can try. Ask your spouse to get involved. Explain to them why this is beneficial to both of you and how important it is to you to have them involved. If they still do not want to, be strong and remember your goals. A lot of times if your spouse sees you motivated and actively improving your own life, they will be interested/motivated to join.

Use your exercise time as "together time." Most couples find it hard to fit in something as simple as talking to each other. Going for a walk around the block after work each day is great physical activity and allows 5-30 min/day of time to reconnect.

Avoid using guilt as a tool to get the stubborn spouse involved. It might seem like a great idea (I have tried it and failed), but your spouse will just grow to hate the activities.

*Physical Activity for You and Your Spouse*

Circuit training is a fast paced, ever changing style to try. Set up five stations. At each station, have a simple exercise set up (for example—walking, jumping jacks, bicep curls, sit-ups, squats). Set the timer for 3 minutes. Each of you is at a different station. Perform the physical activity, and then rotate to the next station when the 3 minutes is up.

**Radom Circuit**
A: squats      B: triceps pushes      C: chin-ups
D: Bike        E: Shoulder External Rotation

**Cardio Circuit**
A: Bike            B: Elliptical      C: Stepper
D: Rowing Machine  E: Treadmill

Team stretching is used in a lot of middle and high school sports. You stretch the other person's hamstrings for 5 minutes, then switch. Alternate as many times as you need to or have time for.

Long walks are a relaxing way to spend time with your spouse. Take your spouse (and pet) on a walk around the neighborhood or development.

*Children*

Kids are a major obstacle for most parents. Depending on the age, these obstacles will vary greatly. Very small children need constant attention. If your kid likes being held, pick them up and walk around the house/apartment for 5-10 min at a time. Do not just sit with them in your lap. Move with them! Rather than sitting on the couch making sure they do not do anything stupid (all children have the inherent desire to try and kill themselves), get down and roll around on the floor with them. Join in on their activities; you would be amazed at how hard it is to keep up with them! There was a fitness guru many years ago that decided to mimic a baby's movements for a whole day. He was unable to! It is a powerful mixture of isometrics, yoga, and static poses.

What activities can you do with your small children?
1. _____
2. _____
3. _____

Teenagers require you to become their personal taxi service at times. While you are sitting waiting for them, as you inevitably will, go for a short walk around their school (inside or out). I have a friend that has a couple of dumbbells in her car that she curls as she walks at her kid's baseball practice. Those 5, 10, 15 minutes waiting for your kids do not have to be wasted. Teenagers tend to create a lot of stress, especially for the caring parent. Physical activity is a great way to reduce teenager-related stress.

What activities can you do while waiting around for your teenager?
1. _____
2. _____
3. _____

*The Home*

Make your home work. There is nothing to say that you have to walk 15 min around a track or on a path. My grandmother has a winding course through her house that takes her all of 45 sec -1 min to complete. She will do this for the 15 min and then rest.

Use the long hallways, stairs, and hills on your property and in your home to your advantage. You may be required to tidy up around your house to clear walk-able paths. Is there a spare room that is the "junk" room? Can it be cleared and used as the new exercise room?

What are some ways you can improve your environment?
1. _____
2. _____
3. _____


*Company*

      Working out alone is boring (for most). Try and involve friends and family into your routine. You can include different people throughout the day. Walk with your spouse for 10 min before work, a friend for 10 min at lunch, and a neighbor for 10 min after work. Be creative. People tend to be more successful and more motivated when they are exercising with someone.

Who are some friends/co-workers that you can involve?
1. _____
2. _____
3. _____
4. _____
5. _____

*Money*

      Money is important unfortunately. Its importance will vary depending on what you already have available.
      The big-ticket item tends to be a gym membership. For those who need to get out of the house and be around other people, the gym is great. The gym offers motivation, competition, people to talk to, guidance, advice, etc. Some businesses offer discounts at local gyms. Insurance companies are starting to reward their participants for daily exercise with reductions in insurance premiums and/or gym memberships. Contact your employer and

insurance company to see what type of offers they provide. Some businesses have gyms in the building to encourage employees to exercise (exercise during the day has been shown to improve productivity and employee satisfaction, less days missed of work)→use them!

If your business and insurance company do not offer deals, it is time to shop around at local gyms.

What do you want in your gym?
1. _____
2. _____
3. _____
4. _____
5. _____

| My responses: | |
|---|---|
| 1. Budget friendly membership fee | 3. Basketball court |
| | 4. Good group classes |
| 2. Treadmills/elliptical | 5. Convenient hours |

Take this list of 5 things and find the gym that best meets your criteria. There are many gym-chains that are available in most places. Make sure you are getting what you want. If you do not, tell them you are taking your business elsewhere.

### Top 10 Questions to ask before signing a gym membership

1. Do you run promotional offers (reduction in membership cost)? I work at a local business, are there any deals for that? Is there a special family rate?
2. A lot of places will waive the "sign-up" fee. Do you?
3. How long is the membership for? What is the penalty if I decide to discontinue my membership before that time?
4. What are your normal business hours?
5. What are your rules regarding guests? Free passes? How many?
6. What classes are offered (and how often)? Is the price included in my membership?

7. Is the gym/pool used by other groups (local sports teams, high schools, etc)? When? Are the basketball courts closed at any other times?
8. Do you have personal trainers on staff? Does it cost extra to utilize their services (personal trainers, strength and conditioning specialists, athletic trainers, certified weight trainers)?
9. Are there times in the day where the equipment is full? Are there waits for machines?
10. What is your newest equipment? Do you have any "trendy" equipment (ie. Kettle bells, suspension bands, etc)?

*Clothing*

Most people think you need designer work-out clothes just to walk around a track at the gym. If you are a person that needs that, put it in your budget. Most people will be able to get away with an old pair of shorts (or sweats), a t-shirt, and sneakers. It is really that simple. Do not make it harder (or more expensive) than it needs to be. The one piece of clothing I would suggest investing in are your sneakers. They are extremely important for your comfort if you will be doing anything on your feet. Most local shoe stores (and even magazines) will have someone you can talk to about the right shoe for your body type and expected level of activity. I see people every week with injuries and/or pain from improper footwear. These aches and pains serve as an easy excuse not to exercise "just today" or "just this week". Do not fall into the trap! A pair of shoes is the one piece of attire worth spending money on.

Minimalist shoes are the new fad. I see people every week with stress fractures in their feet from running in them. My hope is that they fade like every other fad. My suggestion is to find a supportive, well-cushioned shoe to protect your feet.

*Home Gym*

If you are going to be splashing the cash on a gym membership, I do not personally see the need to have a full arsenal of work-out equipment in your home. If you go to the gym most days of the week, your equipment at home will become furniture, not workout equipment. However, if you are someone who will not be joining a gym, investing in some equipment for home will allow you to perform a wider variety of exercises and even provide some motivation. Working out at home can act as a stepping stone for working out at the gym. I would suggest starting small with equipment. Getting some dumbbells of varying weights is a great start and will allow you to do a wide variety of weight training. A soft mat (yoga mat) is a smart purchase to make floor activities more comfortable. Suspension bands are a new piece of exercise equipment that offers a wide variety of whole body exercises. Exercise balls are becoming popular again for core strengthening. They are relatively cheap and help provide some variety to your routine.

| Equipment | Total |
| --- | --- |
| Yoga Mat, 20 lb kettle bell, suspension bands, exercise ball, glider (small rowing machine) | $35 + $35 + $50 + $20 + $145 = $285 for life! |
| Gym Membership | Month ($30-50)/Year ($360-600) |

What equipment do you think you will need?
1. _____
2. _____
3. _____
4. _____
5. _____

*Planning Your Diet*

The planning stage for diet is a little different (and easier in my opinion). There is an overabundance of diet information out there. What you want to do is create a well-balanced selection of foods for yourself. There are many books and thousands of research articles that talk about very specific, strict diets/meal plans. In theory, these will work very well and you are more than welcome to do this if you choose. I would like to caution you however, that diets that require rigid dedication to the plan with little room for enjoyment tend to have a ridiculously high failure rate long-term. Over the next few weeks, do research online, at the store, etc. Educate yourself on what is considered healthy, what vitamins you want in your diet, etc. (I will provide some more information in the diet chapter).

## "Should Haves" for Your Diet

1. Eat whole grains and avoid white bread/white flour.
2. Eat colorful meals. Add color to your diet with fruits and veggies.
3. Variety over same old-same old. Change up your diet; eat different things so you do not get sick of foods.
4. It is ok to have dessert. Do not eat cheesecake every night, but once or twice a month; it is healthy (mentally/behaviorally) to do this. If you starve yourself of sweet things you enjoy, you will only crave them more. When you do finally break down, you'll over eat.
5. Eat different types of foods. Eat pasta, red meat, poultry, fruits, veggies, nuts, legumes, sweets, fatty foods, and foods high in protein. There are important nutrients in all foods. Eating a wide variety insures you get them all.
6. Portion sizes. This could not be more important. You can eat most things and be healthy if you consume the proper portion sizes. Take a small plate of food and eat that first. This will help trick your brain into eating less by thinking you are eating more. A general rule of thumb is that a portion size is about the size of your fist. So if you only want to have one serving of meat at dinner, do not eat half the cow. Eat slowly. Eating slowly will help give you the feeling of fullness while eating less food.
7. Healthy snacks. Where most people knock out a boat load of calories they do not need is with snacks and drinks. Try healthy snacks (yogurt, nuts, and fruits) rather than the greasy kind. Try drinking more water rather than fruit juice/soda.
8. Eat Organic. Yes, it is more expensive, but it is much healthier for you in the long run (less preservatives, etc).
9. Eat in. Eating out a lot increases your intake of sugar, salt, and the bad kinds of fat. Restaurants do this to make the food taste better.
10. Do not overhaul your diet all at once. This leads to long-term failure. If you eat steak and eggs for breakfast every morning, do not switch to nuts and berries the next morning. The carnivore in

you will not appreciate the immediate reversal. Make the switch very gradually over time.

11. Mediterranean foods. All of the new research is supporting Mediterranean foods (fish, oils, etc) for brain function and overall health.

What are healthy foods you already like?
1. _____
2. _____
3. _____

What are some healthy foods you'd be willing to try adding to your normal diet?
1. _____
2. _____
3. _____

How many servings do you eat in one sitting on average?
Meats _____
Fruits/veggies_____
Sweets _____

    Motivation will be explained in much greater detail in the next month. For this month, just brainstorm things that motivate you.

What motivates me?
1. _____
2. _____
3. _____
4. _____
5. _____

<u>Month 1 Checklist</u>

1. Have found time in my schedule to work out ☐

2. Have someone to workout with ☐

3. Have started trying new healthy foods ☐

4. Have equipment and/or gym membership ☐

5. Have set aside money that I will need to succeed ☐

6. Have various exercises I want to try ☐

7. Have a calendar/journal to write everything down in ☐

# **Month 2: Motivation**

*Goal: Set up a system that will motivate you. Do you need rewards? How often? Decide what type of motivation will work best in the short and long term.*

What type of motivation do you think you respond best to?
1. _____
2. _____
3. _____

     I am going to do my best in this section to give you some strategies and suggestions. At the end of the day, this falls on you. There are countless theories and methods proposed on how to motivate people. I think it falls on the shoulders of the individual. Do you want to change? What can you do to encourage yourself to change?

*Scare Tactics*

     Scare tactics have a certain appeal to them. Threats of cancer, early death, etc. have a certain resonance to them. The problem with threats is that everyone has heard them. We are threatened every day not to do this, or eat that. This is especially true for people who are already unhealthy. They have doctors, therapists, family members, friends, etc. telling them to change, "or else". Unfortunately we become numb to the threats.

On the way to get my drivers license, my dad made a detour and took me through the Intensive Care Unit of the hospital to meet a number of paralyzed and dismembered patients and just chat with them. They were all driving related accidents, as I am sure you have already guessed. I can assure you that I always buckle up, drive real slow, and will not drive after even a drop of alcohol has hit my tongue. It worked because I had never been in there before. I did not meet these poor injured people every day for 16 years. It is harder to use this same tactic with health related issues that occur over time. People always say, "I am not that bad" or "I will change before it ever gets that bad". Long story short, scaring doesn't work well with the general population and I would suggest not using that as your primary source of motivation. If people are not afraid of the warning labels printed on every pack of cigarettes threatening, cancer, death, harm to pregnancies, etc., then obviously scare tactics and warnings do very little to motivate people to change in the long run. To have a lasting effect, a true lifestyle change, you have to want to do it.

*Yummy Yummy Food*

A lot of people use food as a reward for exercising a lot and/or sticking with a strict diet. In theory, this is a great idea. In practice, it can hurt you more than help if you are not careful.

What foods do you enjoy eating on a regular basis?
1. _____
2. _____
3. _____
4. _____
5. _____

What foods are your "treats"?
1. _____
2. _____
3. _____
4. _____

If these foods are completely different, we are in good shape. This would mean that you are eating healthier on a daily basis and having your treats only occasionally. If you eat a treat once a week, or better yet, a month, you are doing well. If there is a food that is on both of these lists, we have a couple problems. It means you are more than likely eating too much junk food (as are most Americans). It can also mean that you are treating/rewarding yourself too often. Herein lies the primary problem with using food as a reward. Most people will start by saying, "I can eat out and get a cheesecake once a month if I stick to my new lifestyle plan as a reward". Once a month is fantastic and will do you no long-term harm. In fact, letting yourself splurge occasionally provides motivation and offers a break from a new healthy diet. It will feed your body's (or in most cases, your mind's) craving for fat and sweets. The problem is that most people do not stick to this; once a month quickly becomes once every two weeks, once a week, and so on. If you have the strength and will power, go for it. If you know (and you know who you are) that this can only work for so long, do not even start using food as a reward.

*Entertainment*

What types of entertainment do you enjoy (think music, movies, etc.)?
1. _____
2. _____
3. _____
4. _____
5. _____

     Buying yourself something at the end of each month is a common motivator. I had a patient recently state when she reached 130° of knee flexion, that she was taking $100 to a casino. She had a knee replacement and was struggling with motivating herself to do the work necessary at home to get better. She set this reward up and quickly achieved her goal. I had another patient with a similar surgery that traded in his truck for a tiny sports car that he had wanted all his life. He quickly attained his goals allowing him to comfortably ride in his car. Allowing yourself to spend a little money you normally would not is a good motivational tool (please make sure you have the budget available to do this!).

I rewarded myself with concert tickets. Each month, for the first year I would purchase two concert tickets to local and popular bands. This achieved two purposes. First of all, I had serious motivation to stick with my goals because there was always another concert I wanted to go to. Secondly, by buying the second ticket, I included friends and loved ones in my efforts. If you do this enough, you start associating your exercise accomplishments with the great excitement and feelings from going to concerts (or whatever it is that motivates you!). Obviously, money is a consideration. Do not set this as your reward system if you are not going to follow through. It is not going to take long for you to interest in your goals without any kind of reward!

What are some activities you would want to go to?
1. _____
2. _____
3. _____
4. _____
5. _____

*Putting Your Feet Up*

Breaks can be used as a form of reward. I caution the use of these because they tend to be overused. The other reason this is not the best idea is that this lifestyle change is supposed to be fun. It should be something you want to do, so giving yourself a day off as a reward just seems counterproductive. If used appropriately, the break can be a good idea. Making lifestyle changes are hard and sometimes it helps to have a day off. To avoid the usual pitfalls, try scheduling your breaks ahead of time on a calendar. Fight the urges to take extra breaks or add one here and there. If you are taking Sundays off, stick to it. An excellent thing to do is to have a journal or large calendar to record your activities on. If you did not do anything one day, mark it out with a big "X" to make it clear you did not do anything. It will serve as a great visual cue if you start seeing a lot of big red X's.

What can you do during your days off to make them productive?
1. _____
2. _____
3. _____
4. _____
5. _____

*Clothing*

     Clothing is a popular reward system. It tends to be a more effective reward for women, but can be used for a lot of men. The idea is that at the end of the month, if you have achieved your goals and maintained your goals from the previous month, you buy yourself something. This can be a new pair of shoes, shirt, pants, a manicure, etc. It should be something you want or have wanted and will be excited to have. This is an effective way of improving your self-image, or how you view yourself. If you are working hard at changing your lifestyle and are starting to lose weight, gain muscle, feel better, getting new clothes can add to your newfound confidence and encourage you to continue improving.

     A lot of people just want to reward themselves with things they want. This can be anything from a movie/video game to dinner out. Just like the clothing, it is effective. Just like the clothing, make sure you have it in the budget before you plan on treating yourself with "stuff" every time you meet a goal.

*Intrinsic Strategies*

     The age of blogging and social networking sites has opened a new a relatively un-used opportunity (I have provided a blog to complement information in this book to further assist you→http://smartlife-learninghealth.blogspot.com/). Sometimes it feels good when other people know about your accomplishments and know what you are doing. One way to include everyone and let them know how you are doing is by creating a blog. At the end of each week you do an entry with pictures and stories from your past week, goals you have accomplished, helpful articles you have found etc. This way you can chart your path (and have people follow you). It has the added benefit of helping other people.

They can see how and what you are doing and get motivated or be given some guidance on how to make changes of their own! Recording what you do and when you are doing it can show you just how much you are doing (like the calendar idea earlier). It is harder to kid yourself when everything is written out in front of you. If you like the idea of keeping notes on your progress, but not advertising it, getting a spiral bound notebook or journal can be a way to do that.

The absolute best kind of motivation is also the hardest for a lot of people to muster up enough of. Everyone wants to look better. But you need something at a slightly higher level than that (although looking better always helps). We need to feel good. We need to feel like we have accomplished something. Turn this into a challenge that you are up against. You want to win. You want to feel good at the end of the day everyday. You need internal motivation. You should feel good about your accomplishments. Make getting healthier a challenge that you succeed at daily.

Month 2 Checklist

1. I have an extrinsic reward set up ☐

2. I have a plan for how often/how much for my rewards ☐

3. I am brainstorming good intrinsic rewards to use ☐

This marks the end of the planning stage. My suggestion to you at this time is to make a master calendar. It should have each day laid out as best as you can. Because you have not had a month where you have had to make a major change to your diet or exercise, use this as a learning tool. Today, you can add hypothetical plans in. As you progress through the chapters you can add real things to your master calendar. For example:

| Monday | **Diet:** Breakfast (cereal, banana, water), Lunch (PB & J, yogurt and granola), Snacks (celery, grapes), Dinner (chicken, broccoli, wheat pasta, salad) **Exercise:** 2 mile jog before work, arm weights at lunch, stretching after work **Motivation:** Movie at the end of the week, blog entries **Planning:** Purchase exercise ball to improve core and leg workouts. |
|---|---|
| | YOUR TURN… |
| Tuesday | |
| Wednesday | |
| Thursday | |

|  |  |
|---|---|
| Friday |  |
| Saturday |  |
| Sunday |  |

    The above table is an example of what your plan will look like. We are going to take it step by small step and make sure that you succeed. I would suggest creating a spreadsheet/table on your computer or buying a large calendar or journal that you can fill in every week. It might seem a little tedious now, but it will pay off big in the end.

# **Month 3: Diet**

*Goal: Make the first meal of the day healthy and have healthy snacks during the day.*

We are entering the true "Action" stage of change. You are making a real, tangible change to your life in this month. It is time to "Put up or shut up." The goal above is your primary goal for this month. I am briefly going to talk about nutrition, then go into some options, and finally some suggestions on how to make this goal a reality and a permanent part of your life. Remember, you have the entire month to reach this goal. Start small and work up. Just a quick note before you get started. The diet section is a little long and I do not want you to get bogged down with specifics. I included a little extra only because diet is a big topic right now and I wanted to make sure you knew why you were making the changes I am suggesting. Read the "science stuff" but pay close attention to the lists and illustrations; I think they will help you.

*Nutrition*

What healthy foods do you like already?
1. _____
2. _____
3. _____
4. _____
5. _____

The first thing to do is learn about the foods you are eating. What are you looking for? What do you want to avoid? What do you want more of? What numbers are you looking for in your blood work?

Cholesterol is something that everyone talks about, but few truly understand. Cholesterol is a steroid alcohol found in animals (plants are cholesterol free!). Most cholesterol is synthesized by the liver (about 80%) with the rest coming from eating animal food sources. Lipoproteins are the proteins that carry cholesterol in the blood. The two primary lipoproteins are HDL and LDL (discussed shortly). The bad thing about cholesterol is that the more cholesterol in the blood stream, the more atherosclerotic plaque, and the harder it is for blood to be pumped through the vessel. This is where cholesterol (and other fatty material) builds up and can narrow and harden the blood vessel (a condition called atherosclerosis). This makes it harder for the body to pump blood through these vessels (raising your blood pressure). This becomes a very large problem in the case of heart disease, stroke, and various other cardiovascular diseases. You want your blood to flow freely through your arteries.

Cholesterol is not all bad—you need some. There is a reason your body makes it. Cholesterol is a precursor to bile acids (aid in dietary fat absorption), steroid hormones (made and released by endocrine glands in the body), released in the blood stream and travel to other parts of the body to affect change, part of the myelin sheaths of nerve cells (the insulation which allows normal conduction), and various other glands (adrenal, etc). Cholesterol also plays a significant role in the normal, crucial functioning of cells.

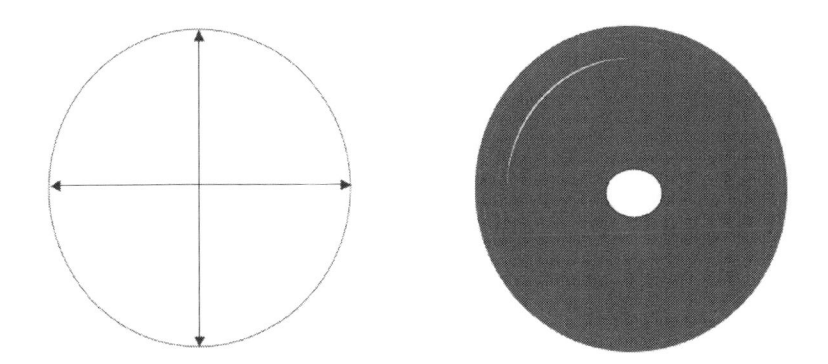

The above image is demonstrating atherosclerosis (when there is too much cholesterol). Just imagine if these vessels were providing blood and nutrients to your heart. The vessel on the left will allow significantly more blood to pass through than the one on the right. When you hear people talking about coronary arteries being occluded, the example on the right is what they are talking about. This significantly reduces the blood getting past this point in the vessel. This is important because blood carries good nutrients (oxygen, hormones, etc) towards areas of the body that need it and take the bad nutrients (carbon dioxide, lactic acid, etc) away for removal. Clogged vessels prevent this normal function from occurring.

HDL (good) and LDL (bad) are both lipoproteins responsible for carrying cholesterol. What they do with the cholesterol is their primary difference and the reason why one is "good" and the other is "bad." HDL's promote the removal of excess cholesterol from the cells out of the body. LDL's pick up cholesterol and drop it in the cells of blood vessels and muscles.

Hopefully the next question is, "How do I increase my HDL and lower my LDL?" There are many ways to increase your HDL's through lifestyle changes and diet. No smoking. Cholesterol should be the least of your worries if you are smoking, but it certainly does not help your cholesterol. Losing weight is helpful. Depending on the source, 25-35% of daily calories should come from fat. Saturated fat should be less than 7% (this is where a lot of people struggle). Along with saturated fats, you are going to want to avoid trans fats. Monounsaturated and polyunsaturated fats (olive/peanut oils) can be a positive part of your diet. Other nuts and fish oils (omega-3) can improve the HDL/LDL ratio. Eat a lot of fiber. As bad as this may sound to some people, drinking alcohol in moderation is also suggested.

*After all of this, what are some foods you should start thinking about?*

Oatmeal, oat bran, high fiber foods, fish and omega-3 fatty acids (halibut, lake trout, salmon, etc), walnuts, almonds, non-salted peanuts, other nuts, olive oil, foods with added plant sterols (yogurt drinks)

---
**Bottom Line:** Keep cholesterol intake to a minimum. Check your nutrition labels and make sure the foods you are eating are low in cholesterol. Eat things high in fiber to help lower your cholesterol.
---

*Triglycerides are something many doctors urge you to keep low. What are they? How do you lower them?*

Triglycerides are the primary type of lipid used for energy storage. When the body gets calories it does not need, they are converted to triglycerides and stored. In other words, if you eat too much (more than you need), it will get stored as fat. It is one of the mechanisms that make yo-yo dieting so undesirable and hard to stop. They can contribute to the hardening and narrowing of vessels as well. High triglycerides can go hand in hand with high LDL and low HDL (not the ratio you want!). Eating healthy and moderate levels of exercise (as for HDL/LDL) are the best ways to reduce your triglycerides.

*I just had blood work but don't know what I'm looking for…*

This is a combination of charts from the American College of Sports Medicine and the American Heart Association.

| **Total Cholesterol** | **Level** |
|---|---|
| Less than 200mg/dL | Desirable |
| 200-239 mg/dL | Borderline high |
| 240 mg/dL + | High |
| **LDL** | **Level** |
| Less than 100 mg/dL | Optimal |
| 100-129 mg/dL | Near optimal |
| 130-159 mg/dL | Borderline high |
| 160-189 mg/dL | High |
| 190 mg/dL | Very high |
| **HDL** | **Level** |
| Less than 40 mg/dL | Low |
| 60 mg/dL + | High (good) |
| **Triglycerides** | **Level** |
| Less than 150 mg/dL | Normal |
| 150-199 mg/dL | Borderline high |
| 200-499 mg/dL | High |
| 500 mg/dL + | Very high |

The bottom line is that you want your total fat intake to be relatively low to reduce the risk of serious disease. Obesity and poor diet will soon overtake smoking as the #1 preventable death in this country. Eat healthy and start exercising.

Most people know fiber is extremely important part of everyone's diet. Where does it come from and how is it used is less commonly known. The good thing is, is that it is very simple!

Fiber is mostly indigestible and comes from plant sources. Insoluble fiber has a laxative function on the digestive process. Soluble fiber dissolves in water and beneficially effects cholesterol (lowers it!) and blood sugar levels. The positive effects on blood sugar levels make it easier to prevent/control diabetes. These effects are extremely important in people who are obese (leading form of malnutrition). These functions help control weight (lowering it). It also serves as fuel for your liver. Fiber helps keep stools soft and waste moving through the digestive tract. It is suggested that an average diet should contain 25-30 grams of fiber per day (some statistics suggest Americans consume less than ½ of that figure). These influences have also been linked to the reduction of gall stones and diverticulitis.

Fiber affects digestion from the moment it enters a person's mouth. It requires food to be chewed more (slows down eating process=feeling more full). It slows digestion/absorption (glucose/sugar enters bloodstream slower=less sugar spikes). The process in which it is dealt with in the colon helps nourish the colon's lining.

*Food Sources high in Fiber*

All-natural cereals, whole-grain bread, fruits, veggies, nuts and seeds, bran (has highest fiber content), brown rice, legumes (beans, lentils, peas), oatmeal, berries, figs, and dietary fiber supplements. Although supplements are helpful, they do not contain all of the important varieties of fiber gained from a well-balanced diet. For this reason, supplements should be taken in adjunct with a well-balanced diet and not in place of one. Surprisingly, fruit juice does not usually contain the fiber richness of their whole fruit origins.

*Versus Low Fiber*

Processed/white foods often have fiber removed. Any white bread/pizza foods are low in fiber.

**Top 10 Common Fiber-filled Foods**
1. Beans
2. Berries
3. Lentils
4. Artichoke
5. Greens (salad, spinach, celery, broccoli etc)
6. Whole Grains, wheat
7. Bran
8. Nuts
9. Squash
10. peas

*Salt*

Salt is a major topic of discussion because of the crucial role it plays in our blood pressure and its overabundance in most foods we eat. High blood pressure, or hypertension, is a major killer all over the world. It is highly prevalent in the United States. This is unfortunate, because in most cases it is highly preventable. At the very least it is manageable. The problem is that it does not have a lot of symptoms (the "silent killer"). Most people do not even know they have high blood pressure unless the doctor tells them so. Anything over 120/80 blood pressure is considered pre-hypertension. At this stage, you need to start making some changes to avoid any damage or progression of the disease. Things like diet and exercise are your first line of defense. 140/90 blood pressure is considered hypertension and you need to consult your doctor on the proper course of action.

Hypertension is a bad thing because it increases your risk of heart attack and stroke. There is new evidence suggesting it can damage your heart, kidneys, brain, and other organs in your body as well.

Salt is important to get into your diet for a normal electrolyte and acid-base balance in your blood. However, too much salt can lead to serious health problems. Salt has the distinction of being highly effective in raising your blood pressure. Added salt can lead to stiff arteries (atherosclerosis discussed earlier), kidney disease, osteoporosis, and left ventricular hypertrophy (where the heart muscle gets larger, in a bad way, to try and pump blood through stiff arteries), among others.

So what does this all mean to you? You must be careful when you are choosing foods to eat. Take-out food, food at restaurants, fast-food, frozen dishes/dinners, and Indian dishes are all extremely high in salt (Why do you think it tastes so good?) and should be limited as much as possible and eliminated when able. Your fruits, veggies, etc are all low in salt. Many foods are also coming out with low-salt or unsalted versions which helps. Make sure to check the nutrition label under "Sodium." The nutrition label will tell you approximately how much of your daily percentage of salt their product will pack in to you.

---

### Top 8 Common Salty Foods
1. Deli meats
2. French fries
3. Bread
4. Chips, pretzels, popcorn
5. Spaghetti/pasta
6. Cheese
7. Canned soups
8. Pizza

**Daily dietary requirements are only approximately 2,300mg of salt. This is only a teaspoon!**

---

*Sugar*

Sugar (carbohydrates) has been the victim of a lot of finger pointing. A gazillion diet plans call for eliminating it completely in all forms (complex and simple carbohydrates). What these diet plans tend to neglect to tell you is that your body MUST HAVE sugar to live. Your brain's sole source of power (is your brain important?) is sugar. The reason for the finger pointing is not because of what sugar is, but what it can do in large amounts. If you eat it in moderation, you will be just fine! The problem is that most foods we eat have an inordinate amount of the stuff in them. Sodas, candy, donuts, refined foods, etc. have a months supply in every bite. In these quantities sugar can be extremely detrimental to your health. Type II diabetes is on the rise and costs the health care system something like ten-million-trillion-billion-gazillion dollars a year and is still rising. Obesity, high cholesterol, high sugar intake, and limited exercise are all significant risk factors for developing type II diabetes. Focusing your carbohydrate intake on complex carbohydrates (whole grains, wheat, multi-grain, bran, etc) is a much healthier alternative to simple/refined sugars and far less harmful to you even in larger quantities. Fruits and veggies contain good sugars as well. Again, inspect your nutrition label for carbohydrates/sugars. Try looking for low calorie/low sugar alternatives if you have to (ideally, without the artificial sweeteners either; which have been linked to cancer).

Sugar is necessary in moderation and harmful in excess quantities. People always ask, "How much is too much?" A simple way to check is to look at the nutrition label and keep track of how many grams of sugar you are getting/day. About half of your calories in a day should be from carbohydrates (explained more later). The nutrition label will give you how much of your daily allowance you are taking in per serving. If the label says carbohydrates………10%; this means when you eat a serving of this food you will have consumed 10% of your daily allowance for carbohydrates. It is also important to note that this is based on a 2,000 calorie day. Depending on who you are and your goals, you may be taking in more or less calories per day and will have to adjust accordingly. The common sense rule can be of service here too. An even simpler way to tell is if you eat white bread, drink soda every day, and enjoy ice cream and other sweets, you are getting too much.

---

**Foods with a lot of Sugar**
1. Canned fruit
2. Canned sauces
3. Pudding
4. Cake
5. Fruit juice/soda
6. Muffins
7. Cereal/cereal bars
8. Ice cream

**Daily dietary requirements are only approximately 20-30 grams!**

---

Before we go any further in our discussion about diet, I would like to address something. I was discussing a few of these topics with my grandmother and she looked at me like I had two heads. "I have made it this far and I am just fine," she said. She does have high cholesterol, hypertension, and emphysema, among other conditions. She believes they are fine because she has medications for them and she is still alive. She also tries to tell me about this friend or that friend that eat nothing but fast food and are "Healthy as a horse." This is a sentiment shared by many of my patients as well. The bottom line is just that some people are plain lucky. Sometimes their genes keep them healthy. However, the grand majority of people are not that lucky and not that genetically inclined. If you wait for it to get so bad that you need medication, damage has already been done and you are now in the business of damage control and rebuilding. Do not wait to act only once it is a problem. Be proactive!

The primary macronutrients are Carbohydrates, Protein, and Fat. Each gram of a specific nutrient contains a specific number of calories:

**1 gram of Carbohydrate has 4 calories**
**1 gram of Protein has 4 calories**
**1 gram of Fat has 9 calories**

Nutrition labels will give you grams of these nutrients. To get the total calories from each nutrient, use the chart above. If there are 10 grams of carbohydrates, multiply it by 4, and you get 40 calories from carbohydrates.

*The Real Deal with Carbohydrates*

Why should you eat carbohydrates? About 45-65% of your total calories should come from carbohydrates, because the main source of fuel used by your body is glucose (carbohydrate/sugar). More specifically, the only source of safe fuel for the brain is carbohydrates. We have not talked much about the brain yet, but trust me, it's important. It is the primary source of fuel, because all tissues/cells can use it. They are important in waste removal and the health of the digestive tract. The primary fuel for any movement/running/exercise lasting less than 90 seconds is from carbohydrates. Think of what you do on a regular basis (at work, etc). Most things last less than 90 seconds, making carbohydrates extremely important to your normal functioning.

*Foods high in Carbohydrates*

Grain, bread, potatoes, cereal, milk, yogurt, fruit/veggies, nuts, beans. Remember from before that fiber is an insoluble carbohydrate (whole grains, fruits/veggies).

> **Weight losing tip:** Celery is high in insoluble fiber and actually has a negative calorie balance. This means that if you eat celery, you are actually losing calories because it takes more energy for the body to try and digest celery than the celery provides!

*Muscle and Cell Building Protein*

Why should you eat protein? About 10-35% of calories should come from protein. Protein is extremely important for growth and immune function. Although it is outside of the scope of the Smart Life Series, protein is also crucial for the production and normal functioning of enzymes and hormones. Protein can be utilized as a fuel source when needed. We will delve into this later as well, but protein is also important in muscle growth, lean muscle, and tissue repair. Every time we lift weights, microscopic tears are caused. These tears are filled/repaired by proteins and eventually lead to muscle hypertrophy (growth).

*Foods high in Protein*

Red meat, chicken, fish, cheese, milk, nuts, legumes (these foods contain the essential amino acids which are the building blocks of all proteins).

*Big Bad Fat*

Why should you eat fat? Isn't fat bad? About 20-35% of calories should come from fat. We want to limit fat in general and even more so for specific types (trans fats, saturated fats), but they are still important to eat. Unsaturated fats (olive oil, avocados, nuts, etc) are the kind you want to focus most of your intake on. Fat is important for normal growth and development. They form the lining of all cells called a lipid bilayer. They are a huge source of energy and can be stored (as most people know all too well).

Vitamins A, D, E, and K are all fat-soluble vitamins. Because these vitamins can be stored for long periods of time, you can get away with eating them less often (less often does not mean the same as never).

### 6 Common Foods Loaded with Fat
1. Meat
2. Dairy
3. Ice cream and other stack foods
4. Fast food
5. Butter, lard, cream
6. Deserts (donuts, cookies, pies, cakes, etc

The next few pages are full of nutritional labels with explanations of the most important things on them! The first is just a blank one for you to familiarize yourself with the layout. Get a box/bag of your favorite food and compare. Find a label from a food you enjoy and write in the empty space below how much "good" and "bad" stuff there is in 1 serving.

### Top 5 Healthy Snacks That Will Actually Cure Hunger Cravings
1. Celery with natural peanut butter and raisins
2. Yogurt, berries, granola
3. Fresh fruit smoothie (fruit, ice, yogurt)
4. Banana and bran muffin
5. Trail mix (unsalted peanuts, pretzels, dark chocolate, raisins)

# NUTRITION FACTS

Serving Size
Servings Per Container

Amount
Per Serving

**Calories**
    Calories from Fat

% **Daily Value** *

**Total Fat**     g
    Saturated Fat     g
    Trans Fat     g
    Polyunsaturated Fat     g
    Monounsaturated Fat     g

**Cholesterol**     mg

**Sodium**     mg

**Potassium**     mg

**Total Carbohydrate**     g
    Dietary Fiber     g
    Soluble Fiber     g
    Insoluble Fiber     g
    Sugars     g

**Protein**     g

Vitamin     ------

* Percent daily values are based on a 2,000 calorie diet. Your daily values may be higher or lower depending on your calorie needs.

How many chips/etc equals a single serving. This is important because all of the numbers below are based on a single serving. If you eat 10 servings, you need to multiply all the numbers below by 10 to see how much you just consumed!

This tells you the total servings in an entire bag. If you eat the entire bag, you must multiply all the numbers below by that total to get your total consumption.

## NUTRITION FACTS

**Serving Size**
**Servings Per Container**

Amount Per Serving

**Calories**
   Calories from Fat

                                        % Daily Value *

**Total Fat**    g
   Saturated Fat   g
   Trans Fat   g
   Polyunsaturated Fat   g
   Monounsaturated Fat   g

**Cholesterol**   mg
**Sodium**   mg
**Potassium**   mg
**Total Carbohydrate**   g
   Dietary Fiber   g
   Soluble Fiber   g
   Insoluble Fiber   g
   Sugars   g
**Protein**   g
Vitamin   -------

* Percent daily values are based on a 2,000 calorie diet. Your daily values may be higher or lower depending on your calorie needs.

If you are monitoring your calories, keep an eye on this number. It does not tell you anything about the real health content or nutrient density, just the total calories. This is commonly where everyone looks first. It is a good place to start, but read on.

This is a slightly more telling sign of the overall healthiness. You want to avoid foods for the most part where the calories from fat make up a high percentage of the total calories. On the whole, you want to limit your total fat intake.

## NUTRITION FACTS

Serving Size
Servings Per Container

Amount
Per Serving

**Calories**

Calories from Fat

% Daily Value *

**Total Fat**         g
   Saturated Fat     g
   Trans Fat         g
   Polyunsaturated Fat   g
   Monounsaturated Fat   g

**Cholesterol**       mg
**Sodium**            mg
**Potassium**         mg
**Total Carbohydrate**   g
   Dietary Fiber     g
   Soluble Fiber     g
   Insoluble Fiber   g
   Sugars            g
**Protein**           g
Vitamin           ------

\* Percent daily values are based on a 2,000 calorie diet. Your daily values may be higher or lower depending on your calorie needs.

| **NUTRITION FACTS** | |
|---|---|
| Serving Size | |
| Servings Per Container | |
| Amount Per Serving | |
| **Calories** | |
| Calories from Fat | |
| | % **Daily Value** * |
| **Total Fat** | g |
| Saturated Fat | g |
| Trans Fat | g |
| Polyunsaturated Fat | g |
| Monounsaturated Fat | g |
| **Cholesterol** | mg |
| **Sodium** | mg |
| **Potassium** | mg |
| **Total Carbohydrate** | g |
| Dietary Fiber | g |
| Soluble Fiber | g |
| Insoluble Fiber | g |
| Sugars | g |
| **Protein** | g |
| Vitamin | ----- |

* Percent daily values are based on a 2,000 calorie diet. Your daily values may be higher or lower depending on your calorie needs.

Does 15g of something give you a good idea of what you are getting? Most people say no and this is where the DV% helps out. These percentages tell you how much one serving contributes to what you are supposed to get all day (based on a 2,000 calorie diet). So if it says 1 serving contains 10% of what you need all day and you eat 3 servings, that means you just consumed 30% of what you need for the whole day for that nutrient.

48

Your grand total in fat for the serving. This number is broken down below to give you a better idea of the types of fat.

The "Bad" fats. These fats lead to atherosclerosis and heart disease. You want these to be as non-existent from your diet as possible.

The "Good" fats. The research currently supports these types of fats as beneficial to you in small amounts. If these make up a high percentage of the total fat content, it is considered OK.

## NUTRITION FACTS

Serving Size
Servings Per Container

Amount
Per Serving

**Calories**
Calories from Fat

% **Daily Value** *

| **Total Fat** | g |
|---|---|
| Saturated Fat | g |
| Trans Fat | g |
| Polyunsaturated Fat | g |
| Monounsaturated Fat | g |
| **Cholesterol** | mg |
| **Sodium** | mg |
| **Potassium** | mg |
| **Total Carbohydrate** | g |
| Dietary Fiber | g |
| Soluble Fiber | g |
| Insoluble Fiber | g |
| Sugars | g |
| **Protein** | g |
| Vitamin | ------ |

* Percent daily values are based on a 2,000 calorie diet. Your daily values may be higher or lower depending on your calorie needs.

You need only very small amounts of cholesterol and salt (sodium) in your diet. Too much can lead to a multitude of heart and health problems. Keep these numbers as low as possible.

## NUTRITION FACTS

Serving Size
Servings Per Container

Amount
Per Serving

**Calories**
    Calories from Fat

% Daily Value *

| | | |
|---|---|---|
| **Total Fat** | g | |
|    Saturated Fat | g | |
|    Trans Fat | g | |
|    Polyunsaturated Fat | g | |
|    Monounsaturated Fat | g | |
| **Cholesterol** | mg | |
| **Sodium** | mg | |
| **Potassium** | mg | |
| **Total Carbohydrate** | g | |
|    Dietary Fiber | g | |
|    Soluble Fiber | g | |
|    Insoluble Fiber | g | |
|    Sugars | g | |
| **Protein** | g | |
| Vitamin | ------ | |

\* Percent daily values are based on a 2,000 calorie diet. Your daily values may be higher or lower depending on your calorie needs.

## NUTRITION FACTS

| | |
|---|---|
| Serving Size | |
| Servings Per Container | |

Amount
Per Serving

**Calories**
   Calories from Fat

**% Daily Value ***

| | | |
|---|---|---|
| **Total Fat** | g | |
|   Saturated Fat | g | |
|   Trans Fat | g | |
|   Polyunsaturated Fat | g | |
|   Monounsaturated Fat | g | |
| **Cholesterol** | mg | |
| **Sodium** | mg | |
| **Potassium** | mg | |
| **Total Carbohydrate** | g | |
|   Dietary Fiber | g | |
|   Soluble Fiber | g | |
|   Insoluble Fiber | g | |
|   Sugars | g | |
| **Protein** | g | |
| Vitamin | ------ | |

*Percent daily values are based on a 2,000 calorie diet. Your daily values may be higher or lower depending on your calorie needs.

Potassium is good for normal health and cellular functioning (including electrolyte balance).

51

| NUTRITION FACTS ||
|---|---|
| Serving Size ||
| Servings Per Container ||
| Amount Per Serving ||
| **Calories** ||
| Calories from Fat ||
| | % Daily Value * |
| **Total Fat** g ||
| Saturated Fat g ||
| Trans Fat g ||
| Polyunsaturated Fat g ||
| Monounsaturated Fat g ||
| **Cholesterol** mg ||
| **Sodium** mg ||
| **Potassium** mg ||
| **Total Carbohydrate** g ||
| Dietary Fiber g ||
| Soluble Fiber g ||
| Insoluble Fiber g ||
| Sugars g ||
| **Protein** g ||
| Vitamin ------ ||
| * Percent daily values are based on a 2,000 calorie diet. Your daily values may be higher or lower depending on your calorie needs. ||

Anywhere from 50-60% of your calories in a day should come from here. Just remember, that it is better if they come from complex/wheat sources.

Great for metabolism, weight loss, digestion, and general health. You want these numbers to be pretty high.

Every American gets way too much of this category. Keep this number as low as you can.

## NUTRITION FACTS

Serving Size
Servings Per Container

Amount
Per Serving

**Calories**

   Calories from Fat

                                                 % Daily Value *

**Total Fat**         g

   Saturated Fat     g

   Trans Fat     g

   Polyunsaturated Fat     g

   Monounsaturated Fat     g

**Cholesterol**     mg

**Sodium**     mg

**Potassium**     mg

**Total Carbohydrate**     g

   Dietary Fiber     g

   Soluble Fiber     g

   Insoluble Fiber     g

   Sugars     g

**Protein**     g

Vitamin     ------

* Percent daily values are based on a 2,000 calorie diet. Your daily values may be higher or lower depending on your calorie needs.

---

*Protein is great for muscle growth and normal cell function.* (annotation pointing to Protein)

*This section varies greatly depending on how many/what kind of vitamins are present. You want higher numbers here.* (annotation pointing to Vitamin)

*Organization & Suggestions*

Now that you have some background, let us organize things.

What are some foods you need to get more of?
1. _____
2. _____
3. _____
4. _____
5. _____

What are some foods you need to reduce in your diet?
1. _____
2. _____
3. _____
4. _____
5. _____

    Now that we know what we are looking for and what we need to eliminate, let us get started. The goal of this month is to eat a healthy breakfast daily and eat healthier snacks.

What are you eating for breakfast on a regular basis?
1. _____
2. _____
3. _____
4. _____
5. _____

    Look at this list and pick 2 things you can do without. Now replace them with a food you know you need more of.

> **Say your breakfast includes**: Eggs, sausages, bacon, coffee, and hash browns. You decide you need the coffee to function, the eggs and hash browns to feel full, but you can do without the sausages and bacon. A banana and some grapes are a great way to improve your breakfast.

**Do you get fast food in the morning? YES   NO**

What are some healthier options you can have?
1. _____
2. _____
3. _____
4. _____
5. _____

    As with everything in this book, change should be gradual. Only replace a couple items in your normal breakfast initially. Replace them with healthy options you know you like (or at least do not hate). Over the course of the month slowly remove all of the unhealthy elements and replace them with healthy foods. If you need to move even slower, choose 3 days of the week to make these changes, and continue as before for the other 4. Work your way up to all 7 days, then all healthy snacks!

    For those of you who think you have no time to make yourself breakfast and you "have" to go through a drive-thru somewhere, stop and think. How much time does it take to pour a glass of orange juice and eat a banana and granola bar? I just timed it, it took me 5 minutes at a relaxed pace with some reading thrown in. There are many good options for things you can take and eat when you get to work (depending on your job) including: bananas, granola bars, protein bars, oranges, a small cup of grapes, etc. Again, start doing these changes a couple times a week and work your way up to eliminating the drive-thru from your routine. Start preparing/planning your breakfast the night before. Fill your car mug with fruit juice or water, have a granola bar and banana sitting next to your car keys the night before.

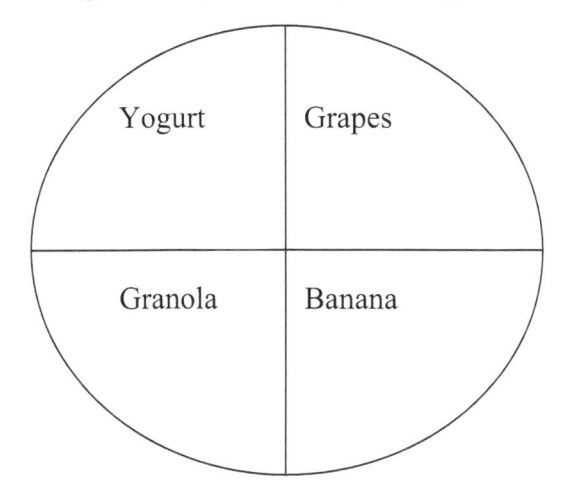

| Yogurt | Grapes |
|--------|--------|
| Granola | Banana |

The diagram shows what an average breakfast plate will hopefully look like by the end of the month. Obviously, these are not your only options, you are the boss! Remember to eat a breakfast, even a small one. If you have not had food since the night before, 9PM?, then your body is starting to wonder when will it get food again? If you skip breakfast and wait for lunch, your body will enter starvation mode. Your metabolism will be slower and by the time you eat, your body is prepared to put almost everything in storage (the nice way of saying fat) in case you try to starve it again.

The other part of our primary goal is to have healthier snacks throughout the day. Many people enjoy chips, another quick run through the drive-thru, or a trip to the vending machine for something equally bad for your body. More than anything, this takes a little planning. You need something that is easy to carry and will fill you up in a pinch. Personally, my solution has been trail mix. I have a big bucket of it in the pantry with lightly salted pretzels, unsalted peanuts, whole grain cereal, raisins, and the occasional piece of chocolate. You are going to want something easy to grab and something that won't spoil throughout the day. Grapes, cucumbers, carrots, etc., usually need some way of keeping cool. Bananas and apples are easy fruits to bring. I personally need that full feeling sometimes, hence the peanuts. Nuts in general are a good snack to keep you going. Keep it simple. The more complex and time consuming the snack gets, the lower the chances you will actually follow through with it.

The following table was created to give you a quick reference to common foods. It gives you the most important information you need to know when selecting these foods. I am hoping it will help you make healthier diet decisions, especially early on. All the information on the table is given based on 1 serving (as per USDA). Keep in mind that one serving of green beans might be a cup, but fried chicken might be 1 piece. They are listed in alphabetical order. Please also be aware that the way you prepare these foods will have an impact on all these statistics as well.

| Food | Total Calories | Fat Content (%DV) | Reason why you should eat it (or not). |
|---|---|---|---|
| Apples | 65 | 0 % | High fiber, vit C |
| Apricot | 74 | 1 % | High fiber, vit C/A, iron, potassium |
| Asparagus | 27 | 0% | High fiber, vit k, iron |
| Banana | 200 | 1% | High fiber, Vit C/B6, potassium |
| Blackberries | 62 | 1% | High vit C/K, fiber, manganese |
| Blueberries | 84 | 1% | High vit C/K, fiber, manganese |
| Bread (wheat) | 66 | 1% | High calcium, manganese, iron |
| Bread (white) | 165 | 1% | High sodium |
| Broccoli | 31 | 1% | High vit C/K/A, fiber, folate |
| Cantaloupe | 60 | 1% | High vit A/C, potassium |
| Carrots | 52 | 0% | High fiber, vit A/K |
| Celery | 18 | 0% | High fiber, vit A/K |
| Cheese (cheddar) | 532 | 67% | High calcium, sat fat, cholesterol, sodium |
| Chicken (grilled) | 231 | 8% | High in protein and cholesterol |
| Chicken (fried) | 809 | 75% | High in all types of fat |
| Chicken (nugget) | 83 | 9% | High in fat, cholesterol, sodium |
| Chickpeas | 269 | 7% | High fiber, iron |
| Coffee | 2 | 0% | Some riboflavin |

| | | | |
|---|---|---|---|
| Cucumber | 8 | 0% | High vit K |
| Egg (whole) | 211 | 22% | High cholesterol, protein |
| French fries | 539 | 44% | High in all types of fat, cholesterol |
| French Toast | 149 | 11% | High in fat, cholesterol, sodium |
| Grapes | 104 | 0% | High vit C/K |
| Green beans | 34 | 0% | High fiber, vit A/C/K, folate |
| Hamburger (plain) | 216 | 22% | High in fat, cholesterol, iron |
| Honey | 85 | 0% | High in sugar |
| Kiwi | 108 | 1% | High in fiber and vit C/K, potassium, folate |
| Lettuce (romaine) | 1 | 0% | High vit A |
| Mango | 107 | 1% | High fiber, vit A/K/B6 |
| Milk (whole) | 146 | 12% | High in sat fat, cholesterol, calcium, vit D |
| Mushrooms | 15 | 0% | High riboflavin and niacin |
| Nectarine | 63 | 1% | High fiber, vit A/C, niacin |
| Nuts/almonds | 167 | 23% | High magnesium, vit E, manganese |
| Oil (olive) | 248 | 43% | High mono/poly unsat fats, omega-fatty acids (good for you!) |
| Onions | 64 | 0% | High fiber, vit B6, folate, potassium, manganese |

| | | | |
|---|---|---|---|
| Oranges | 85 | 1% | High fiber, vit C |
| Pancakes | 175 | 11% | High cholesterol, sodium, carbs |
| Pears | 86 | 0% | High fiber, vit K |
| Pineapple | 74 | 0% | High thiamin, vit B6/C |
| Plums | 76 | 1% | High vit A/C |
| Potatoes (baked) | 174 | 1% | High carbs, iron, vit B6 |
| Potatoes (Mashed with butter) | 278 | 2% | High vit C, fiber |
| Rice (brown) | 216 | 3% | High selenium and manganese |
| Salmon | 159 | 9% | High niacin, vit B6/12, phosphorus, protein |
| Seeds (flaxseed) | 150 | 18% | High in thiamin, magnesium, phosphorus, copper, manganese |
| Shrimp | 84 | 1% | High iron, selenium, phosphorus |
| Snap peas | 41 | 0% | High riboflavin, vit B6, pantothenic acid, fiber, folate |
| Spaghetti | 221 | 2% | High thiamin, folate, selenium |
| Spinach | 7 | 0% | High vit A/C/K, folate, manganese, iron |
| Squash | 18 | 0% | High protein, vit A/K, thiamin, niacin, copper |
| Strawberries | 49 | 1% | High vit C, |

| Strawberries | | | manganese, folate |
|---|---|---|---|
| Steak | 1,116 | 95% | High cholesterol, sat fat, protein |
| Sweet Potato | 180 | 0% | High vit A/C, fiber, iron |
| Tomatoes | 27 | 0% | High vit E/B6, thiamin, niacin, fiber |
| Quinoa | 103 | 3% | High folate, magnesium, phosphorus |

## Month 3 Checklist

1. I eat a healthy breakfast every day of the week. ☐
2. I leave out healthy snacks for the next day before I go to bed. ☐
3. I have healthy snacks each day. ☐

# Month 4: Cardio

*Goal: By the end of the month you will perform 30 minutes of cardiovascular exercise 3 out of 7 days in the week.*

Not many people enjoy cardiovascular exercise. Most people come up with a wide variety of excuses not to do it. Unfortunately, it is one of the single most important things you can do for every aspect of your health. It literally has the ability to prolong your life.

*Background on the Heart, Lungs, and Circulation*

I am going to attempt not to bore you, but I think that it is important to have some understanding of what is going on in your body.

To put it lightly, the heart is super-duper-extra-mega-important. It is responsible for taking blood in, sending it to the lungs, and then spreading it throughout the entire body to the very tips of every part of your body.

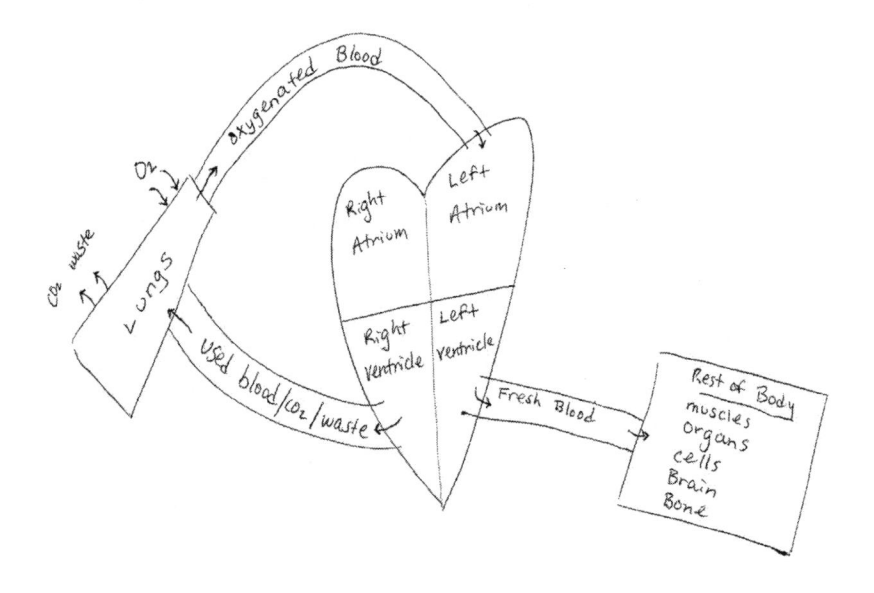

It takes in what I call "used blood", or blood that is depleted of oxygen and loaded up with waste (mainly carbon dioxide). There is a valve in the middle of the heart that sends all of this blood to the lungs where the carbon dioxide is breathed out and the red blood cells pick up the new oxygen you just breathed in. This blood is brought into the heart through a separate valve and this side of the heart then sends the blood out of the heart completely. This "fresh" blood travels through the arteries in your body and delivers all of the life-sustaining nutrients and oxygen to the working tissues in the body (bones, brain, muscle, etc).

When you exercise, the demand for blood and nutrients (like oxygen) goes up significantly. Even when you move from a seated position to a standing one there is an increased demand by the gluteal (butt) muscles that help you stand up. Your body needs to be able to respond. In some cases, you will need to work up to this point. Your heart currently has a limit of blood and oxygen it can circulate. By training, you can increase the capacity of your heart to work. You can actually reduce your heart rate and pump out more blood. How? Your heart gets stronger and is able to pump more blood every time. Remember that your brain likes getting blood and oxygen too. You want to have a cardiopulmonary system that is going to be very efficient at this task. This is hugely beneficial to your overall health and your quality of life.

Each time it beats, the heart needs to get as much blood out to your working body as your body demands. If you can barely stand up and go to the bathroom or refrigerator without getting short of breath and/or tired, how much quality of life will you have? How will you be able to participate in hobbies, play with your children or grandchildren, or walk around the grocery store without a motor?

The more you perform cardiovascular exercises, the more efficient this system becomes and the healthier you become.

*Benefits*

What do you think are some benefits of cardio exercise?
1. _____
2. _____
3. _____
4. _____
5. _____


The following are a small sampling of important benefits:

Performing cardiovascular exercise on a regular basis will increase your metabolism. This means your body will burn more calories during a normal day (during the actual exercise and after you have stopped!). An increased metabolism will lead to decreased weight.

Regular cardio will decrease your risk of heart disease, heart attack, coronary artery disease, stroke, etc. A lot of these diseases involve an artery getting clogged up by fatty plaques (atherosclerosis). Thousands of people every year require stents to open up "blocked arteries" so their heart gets the blood it needs. When the heart stops pumping blood, your body does not get the constant flow of nutrients it requires and bad things happen. Performing regular cardio will help open up and keep your arteries clear. Cardio trains the heart to pump more blood out with less effort. It allows a more constant, non-interrupted flow of nutrients.

You could spend years talking about the heart, lung, and vascular benefits of cardio exercise, but Iwill spare you the time and just tell you it is REALLY important and does AMAZING things for your cardiopulmonary and cardiovascular system.

The benefits for the arteries around the heart, lungs, and brain extend to the whole body. Arteries all over the body become stronger and wider (by preventing fatty plaque build-up) to allow for the increased flow of blood to tissues in constant need. Cardio exercise significantly reduces the risk of atherosclerosis and has even been shown to help reverse it to some degree.

Cardiovascular exercise has been proven to improve self-management of diabetes. Cardio exercise increases the body's sensitivity to insulin and will decrease your blood sugar levels. If started early enough and performed routinely enough, people can stop taking their medications because the cardio is controlling their blood sugar levels (consult your physician before making any changes to your medications!!).

Cardiovascular exercise has been shown to reduce stress levels and improve mood. Longer, sustained exercise bouts will have more substantial effects, but you will see improvements even with minimal activity. When you perform this type of physical activity your body will release endorphins (causing the runner's high) and make you feel good.

Cardiovascular exercise is important in increasing bone mineral density (stronger bones). The repetitive stress, especially on your legs, causes the bones to bulk up to withstand the impacts.

During cardiovascular exercise your blood pressure will rise based on how hard you are working out. The real benefit comes later. After exercising for a while, your blood pressure will actually go down at rest. This means that your heart will be beating against less resistance (which means better blood flow and less work for the heart). Once again, with the proper type and amount of cardio, people can actually get off of their expensive blood pressure medications because they have learned to control it with exercise (please consult your physician before making any changes to your medication!!).

Part of the reason your blood pressure is decreased is that you lower the amount of fat in your body. This lowers cholesterol, triglycerides, and the risk of atherosclerosis (clogged arteries). At low to moderate levels of cardio activity, your body will burn mostly fat calories. Have a little padding around your midsection or thighs? Doing crunches every day will not do the trick. Doing crunches is great and you will build strong abdominal muscles. However, until the fat around your belly is gone, you will not see them! You need to get rid of that fat and the way to do it is through prolonged cardiovascular exercise.

Believe it or not, exercising will actually increase your energy levels throughout the day. A lot of people think it will wipe them out and avoid it because they do not want to be too tired the rest of the day. Doing routine cardio will make your body stronger and more efficient. This allows your body to spend less energy and effort doing routine tasks, leaving you loads of energy to spend. Due to this extra energy, it is reported that your energy for other activities and experiences will improve—your sex life gets better!

Not to sound contradictory, but it also helps you get to sleep. After a high energy day with lots of activity, your body will want to recover. It does not mean you will be tired all day. It does mean that you will have a sounder sleep. My brothers both have a torrid time getting any sleep at night. They have found that if they are highly active all day and complete good workouts, then they fall asleep more easily.

As we get older, our joints break down. Usually this is because we lose fluid as we get older. The discs in our back and the fluids in our joints dry up. There is no way to prevent it, but we can do a significant job delaying and slowing it down. Routine cardio requires lots of fluid/smooth joint movements which encourages the fluid to stay in the joints. This leads to improved joint mobility and reduced joint pain.

The same constant and smooth motion that improves joint mobility also leads to improved flexibility. When you use your muscles they warm up and relax. This is why most research suggests doing a small warm-up instead of stretching before activity. Think of your muscles like a rubber band. If you stretch it cold, it is hard and runs the risk of damage. If instead, you lightly move it around, it will warm up and loosen up and become very malleable and stretchy. The same holds true for your muscles.

Cardiovascular exercise improves digestion. This improved digestion leads to a reduced risk of colon cancer.

Teamed with a healthy, high fiber diet, cardio can significantly reduce your risk of developing colon (and other forms) cancer.

More and more research is now suggesting that cardio can reduce the risk of developing Parkinson's and Alzheimer's disease. Obviously cardio does not make you immune to these diseases, but it may reduce your risk. The research is not clear on any direct links; they are just noticing strong correlations. For people who already have these diseases, cardiovascular exercise is a crucial part of maintaining a quality of life. Cardio will improve your breathing ability and capacity to move around. It is imperative that you include cardiovascular exercise into your life even after being diagnosed. All of the above reasons still hold true, specifically (and more importantly) the pulmonary (breathing) and mobility examples.

The above list could be pages upon pages of various benefits ranging from the cellular to spiritual level. In case it hasn't sunk in…CARDIO IS IMPORTANT.

| **What is Cardio good for again?** |
| --- |
| 1. Increased metabolism |
| 2. Decreased risk of heart disease, heart attack, stroke, etc |
| 3. Increased pulmonary function (breathing) |
| 4. Improved self-management of diabetes |
| 5. Reduced stress levels |
| 6. Increased bone mineral density (stronger bones) |
| 7. Decreased blood pressure |
| 8. Decreased cholesterol and triglycerides |
| 9. Increased energy levels |
| 10. Improved sleep |
| 11. Improved joint function |
| 12. Improved digestion |

*Where is the time?*

If people have progressed smoothly through the first three months, this is generally where difficulties start to arise. Not many people like getting sweaty and tired. Some people feel they cannot set aside that much time in their day.

Fortunately, research has shown that exercise can be done in 10-minute increments as long as they add up to 30 minutes by the end of the day. 10 minutes of moderate activity, 3 times a day is your goal. You do not have to get sweaty and dirty or set aside a whole day just to fit in some cardiovascular exercise. "Moderate" activity can range from walking to football depending on your current fitness level (you determine the level). The goal is to raise your breath and heart rate and keep it up for at least ten minutes at a time.

I have created the "Tired Rule" as a general guiding principal for you. If at the end of your cardio activity (the 30 minute total) you are physically tired, then you have done enough. If at the end of your cardio for the day, you feel like you can still run a marathon, you need to think about challenging yourself more from now on. As you get more used to this, try doing two sessions of fifteen minutes. By the end of the year, you should get a whole thirty minutes (or more) in during one session! Watch out; you might just enjoy it.

What parts of the day can you sneak in ten minutes for cardio?
1. _____
2. _____
3. _____
4. _____
5. _____

---

**Tips for sneaking in ten minutes**

1. Set your alarm slightly ahead and get a quick work out in before your morning shower.
2. Take ten minutes out of your lunch.
3. Ten minutes right after you get home from work before you do anything else.
4. If you shower in the evening, exercise ten minutes right before your shower.

---

*How to: Styles and Concepts*

Your focus here should be to achieve a good well-rounded routine. Athletes are always looking to improve a very specific aspect of their game; you just want to improve everything a little bit. Your goal will be to improve your ability to pump blood and take in oxygen. This can mean walking, running, mountain climbing, and bike racing, whatever you want. Ideally, you will do a little bit of everything.

You have both aerobic and anaerobic pathways in your body. The aerobic pathway produces energy by using oxygen. The anaerobic pathway produces energy without oxygen. To sprint (or lift weights) or do bursts of energy less than a minute, we use the anaerobic pathway. A major limitation to this pathway is the available time our body can produce energy without oxygen. A side effect of this type of exercise is the build-up of lactic acid (the burn you feel). Once we have used up our anaerobic stores, we need to rely on other pathways or wait for the anaerobic stores to refill. This pathway is trainable. The more sprints and high intensity activities you do, the better your body becomes at producing energy, increasing stores, and removing lactic acid. It might seem pointless to train this for your everyday life, but it can come in handy in tight situations (running away from something, climbing stairs, etc). When you think about it, there are a lot of situations involving this pathway (lasting less than a minute): Standing up, going up and down stairs, getting in/out of a car, helping carry a heavy object, closing a door, etc.

The aerobic pathway is our main focus. We want to train our body to more efficiently take oxygen from the air, put it in the blood, and deliver it to the necessary tissue as quickly and easily as possible. To do this we need to perform longer sessions of exercise (greater than 1 minute, closer to 10 or more minutes is preferable).

How do we train these different pathways? We follow the specificity and SAID (specific adaptations to imposed demands) principles. All they say is that if you want to improve high intensity pathways, perform high intensity activities. If you want your cardiovascular system to be able to pump so much blood and oxygen over a 15 minute period, try performing activities for 15 minutes or more at a time to train that pathway. If all you do are short 10 yards sprints once a minute every 15 minutes, you will get minimal aerobic benefits because this is an anaerobic (high intensity exercise). You will make anaerobic gains. Train what you hope to improve.

How do you track your progress? How do you know you are improving? There are a couple ways. You can monitor your heart rate (check your pulse). As you become more cardiovascularly trained, your heart rate will decrease. Your heart rate should decrease at rest and go up less during exercise. If you run a mile on day 1 and your heart rate is 120, then on day 30 when you run a mile at the same pace on the same course, your heart rate should be lower (sign of aerobic improvement). Another easy way is the time test. If you can run a 100 yard sprint in 30 seconds the first day, but are running it in 25 seconds on day 30, yo have improved your anaerobic system (same holds true for the aerobic system and long runs). Distance is an easy way to track progress. How far can you sprint or jog before feeling tired? This distance should increase as you train. Finally, how easy was it? If running a mile used to wipe you out and now you are only mildly out of breath, you are improving.

Having some variety in your routine is important both mentally and physically. Mentally, you need a change every once in a while. If you get on the same bike for 30 minutes each day, sooner or later, it will be incredibly boring. If you are set and happy on only one activity (like the bike), vary your intensity. One workout sprint 10 times in the middle, on another maintain a moderate pace the whole time. Change it up. Physically it is good to place different demands on the body. You want to improve all aspects of your cardiovascular fitness. Include sprints some days, longer lighter sessions other days. This allows you to stress both the anaerobic and aerobic systems and improve them.

**Variety Example**
*Monday*: Bike 30 minutes at a moderate intensity
*Tuesday*: Bike 15 min at light pace, 10 at intense pace, 5 min at moderate pace.
*Wednesday*: Rowing machine for 20 minutes, elliptical for 10 min.
*Thursday*: Rowing machine for 30 minutes total. Sprint the first 15 seconds of every minute.
*Friday*: Bike 5 min, row 20 min, elliptical 5 min at high intensity

A lot of athletes use cross training as a way to stay in shape during an off-season without burning out. Eventually, your body needs a break from the same routine. If you run for 6 months straight and that is your only form of cardio, take a month or two off and try a different activity (swimming, rowing, hiking etc.).

How long should I go? Can I take a break? If you are going at a moderate pace, my suggestion would be to take as few breaks as possible to gain maximal cardiovascular benefit. However, if you need a quick breather and a drink, take it. Remember, doing 10 minute intervals 3 times during the day has the same benefit as one 30 minute session. The longer you can maintain an elevated heart rate, the more benefit you will get. If you are not up to that level and you can only do 3 minutes at a time, that is fine! Remember, everything is at your own pace.

*The Bottom Line*

A lot of people take the information from the past few pages and set up complex workouts and time tables. They want to challenge various physiological pathways and stress this or that system in different ways. Keep it simple. You are not training for the Olympics (if you are, you might want to invest in a different book). Get your cardio in any way you can and be done with it. The next few pages can act as your cardio journal for a while if you do not already have one. If you do already have one, maybe use these tables as week totals. It may be interesting to see how you are doing from week to week.

A lot of people suffer from aching joints, arthritis, etc. The table below will give you an idea of what type of activities to choose from. The no-impact column shows exercises that are kindest to your aching joints, all the way to high impact which are best done once you have been exercising a little while longer. If you do have aching joints, consider working out on softer surfaces when possible. If you want to walk, try finding grass to walk on rather than pavement. Be smart about this. If it hurts, look for a lower impact alternative.

| No-Impact | Low-Impact | Med-Impact | High-Impact |
|---|---|---|---|
| Bicycling | Walking | Jogging (slow) | Jogging (fast) |
| Rowing | Stair-Stepper | Jumping Rope | Running |
| Kayaking | NordicTrak | | Plyometrics |
| Swimming | Elliptical | | Soccer |
| Arm bike | | | Football |
| Chair aerobics | | | Basketball |
| Water aerobics | | | |

| Date | Total Time | Activity | Feelings |
|---|---|---|---|
| 3-30-11<br>4-2-11<br>4-4-11 | 45 (all AM) | Bike, Row | Negative before, content after |
|  |  |  |  |
|  |  |  |  |
|  |  |  |  |
|  |  |  |  |
|  |  |  |  |
|  |  |  |  |
|  |  |  |  |
|  |  |  |  |
|  |  |  |  |
|  |  |  |  |
|  |  |  |  |

*Obesity*

     Obesity is an ever-growing problem in the world. People are trying all sorts of things to prevent it and/or control it. It has become so bad that over a third of children are overweight now and as many as two-thirds of adults are. Along with eating healthy and lifting weights, I feel that cardiovascular exercise is the most important factor. I understand that there are many factors that go into the obesity epidemic, but from what I have seen, cardiovascular exercise is the key. Cardiovascular exercise can help significantly lower body weight (do you see many overweight cross-country runners?). The lowering of body weight (and increased cardiovascular exercise) reduces the risk of heart problems and can control diabetes (Type II specifically) without medication (in addition to everything listed earlier in the chapter).

Even if pounds of body weight do not immediately come pouring off, it is still hugely beneficial. You will still see heart benefits, reduced chronic diseases, and improved mental well-being. It is also important to note here that lean muscle mass (your muscles) weigh more than fat. So you can actually reduce the amount of fat and not actually lose any weight. This is ok! A friend on my routine just commented on the fact that he is still stuck at 192, but he needs to wear a belt with his pants now or they fall down. His weight is the same (which had him discouraged), but he is thinning out already. He is just in the fourth month and he is already seeing noticeable progress!

Month 4 Checklist
1. I have the necessary equipment or gym membership to succeed in my goals ☐
2. I am currently performing at least 30 minutes of cardiovascular exercise throughout the day 3 out of 7 days in the week ☐
3. My schedule is arranged well so that I am able to fit in my cardio exercise easily without adding stress to my day ☐
4. I have activities that I enjoy doing daily ☐

# Month 5: Resistance

*Goal: By the end of the month you will perform 30 minutes of resistance exercise 3 out of 7 days in the week.*

Resistance training and weight lifting are usually synonymous, but do not have to be. Resistance exercises just involve you moving your body, or part of your body, against some resistance—simple right? It can be as small as the force of gravity (which can be significant). Most people picture resistance training as going to a large gym and lifting enormous hunks of iron up over your head. In reality, it just involves you moving a body part against something that is above what is normally required of that body part.

*Background on Muscle and Nerves*

Each muscle is actually a group of muscle fibers bundled together. When you want to lift something, make that muscle contract, your brain sends a signal down to the muscle and stimulates as much of the muscle as it needs to perform that task. If you are lifting only the weight of your arm, only a small percentage of your muscle will contract to get the job done. If you lift a really heavy weight, your body will recruit every last bit of the muscle and any muscles around it that might help, to lift that weight. This is an important concept for us. If one of your goals is to build muscle, then you will have to lift something heavy enough to make you tired. If you only lift light weights, your body does not have to try very hard to get the job done. Lifting light weights/high repetitions every day will not build up your strength nearly as much as lifting very heavy weights/low repetitions. You can actually train more nerves to be involved in the contraction of a muscle. If you are constantly lifting heavy weights and trying really hard to accomplish something, more nerves need to be recruited to make more fibers contract. By stimulating more nerve fibers to fire, you will notice significant gains in your muscle strength before you ever see your muscles grow. If you continue to lift heavier and heavier weights, you will see improvements in your muscle size as well. If your goal is endurance and not strength, the low weight/high repetition route will be best for you. The downside with this path is that you will not get nearly the same amount of benefits from strength and resistance training as you would from high weight/low repetition activities.

*Benefits*

Resistance training leads to improved bone mineral density (stronger bones). Lifting weights puts an increased stress on your bones (specifically the involved ones). Your bones respond to this stress by making themselves stronger to avoid any injury (just as your muscles and cardiovascular system do). Increased bone strength prevents fractures, osteoporosis, etc. Especially as you get older, bone strength becomes crucial. A significant portion of elderly people who fracture their hip, die in the 1st year after the injury. A fracture in frail individuals is a long recovery process that some never succeed in. By around age 35 your body stops increasing bone density and you lose a little every year. For this reason we want to build up our bone stores as much as possible before that time. If you are older, do not think there is no point now. Doing regular resistance training greatly reduces the speed at which you lose bone density and some people argue you can bring that process almost to a halt (and maybe even reverse it). Stronger bones will allow you to have a greater quality of life as you get older.

The most obvious result of resistance training is that you get stronger. Strength is important as it allows you to interact in more ways with your environment safely. Being stronger allows you to do more around your own home and recreationally. It opens up all sorts of doors for you. You can do more for yourself without the aid of other people or machines. It gives you far more independence as you get older and reduces the risk of common injuries (falls, tears, etc).

Muscle mass has a faster metabolism than fat does. By increasing the amount of muscle mass you have, you can accelerate your metabolism (burn more calories) during and after exercise and lose weight and fat mass.

Improved mobility is huge. This is obviously more of an issue as you age, but holds true throughout the entire lifespan. Being stronger helps you improve balance. People are more comfortable on their feet with increased strength. You are able to stand up, lie down, and move around with far greater ease and far less effort with more strength. It makes the usual every day activities easy and not exhausting.

❖

One thing I would like to make clear before we go any further—there is no such thing as spot reduction. Spot reduction is the belief that you can do 200 crunches a day and lose weight around your stomach. This is just not true. You will build muscle in your stomach, but not lose weight right there. You may improve your metabolism and globally start to lose weight, just not specifically in that spot. For this reason, do not bother with those electric belts. If your abs are under a thick layer of fat, no amount of time with one of those belts on will give you the fake abs shown in the commercials. As your fat (all over your body) reduces, you will be able to tone certain areas (increase muscle). Put in the real work—diet, cardio, and resistance training.

❖

*Where is the time?*

At this point, you have found 30 minutes, 3x/week to perform cardiovascular exercise. My suggestion would be to perform resistance training on the days you are not doing your cardio. Take the same times each day and just do resistance. If you are doing 20 minutes before work and 10 minutes of cardio immediately after on Monday/Wednesday/Friday, introduce 20 minutes before/10 after on Tuesday/Thursday/Saturday for resistance. This will help you get into a more regular daily routine of some kind of exercise or another. It will allow you to slowly carve parts of your day out for routine exercise. Another option would be to do your cardio immediately before work and your resistance 30 minutes immediately after on the 3 same days of the week. This will give you rest days in between. I would only caution that if you have not exercised much before, this may really make you tired and increase your risk of overuse injury initially. It also robs you of getting into a truly daily routine (which you will be doing eventually anyway!).

*The Whole Body*

This program was not developed for athletes; therefore, we do not have a small group of specific muscles we need to train. We want to train the whole body for overall wellness. The first mistake people make is wanting to train the "look at me" muscles (biceps, pecs, calves). These might be nice to look at and we will train them, but as far as your general health and reduction of injuries, we are going to want to train everything (front/back of legs, entire trunk, front/back of arms, neck).

*How to Workout*

Just like cardiovascular exercise, the goal is to get a total of 30 minutes in a day, but can be done in 10-minute increments. Everyone is concerned about how many sets/reps/weight. Generally, I tell patients 2 sets of 15 repetitions or 3 sets of 7-10. The truth is, you should do enough repetitions and weight to make you tired at the end. If you do 3,000 bicep curls and you do not feel in the least bit tired, you need to increase the weight significantly. For strength gains, do not do more than 15 repetitions in a set. You are starting to work more endurance than strength after that point. If it is really easy to do 15, increase your resistance. At the end of every set, the last repetition you do should be the last possible one you can do with proper form ("sets to exhaustion"). Proper form is key. If you start doing repetitions with terrible form you run the risk of injuring yourself (and you get less out of it anyway). If you have done a good workout, you will have mildly sore muscles the next day.

To improve muscle mass (if you want to see your muscles grow), the general thought is to increase total volume (weight x reps). It is important to note that you will see significant improvements in strength very soon without seeing a large increase in the size of your muscles. Neurologic changes occur first and account for the strength improvements initially. In other words, do 2-3 sets of 5-10 repetitions of a specific exercise. At the end of that, you should be seriously fatigued for whatever muscle you were using. I have found that, especially in beginners, the 2 sets of 15 rule works well as long as there is enough weight lifted to fatigue the muscles.

> **Sample Week**
> 1. *Monday*: 3 sets of 8 reps for the upper body.
> 2. *Tuesday*: 4 sets of 20 reps of core exercises. 2 sets of 8 reps for the lower body.
> 3. *Wednesday*: OFF
> 4. *Thursday*: 3 sets of 20 reps for the upper body. 3 sets of 20 reps of core exercises.
> 5. *Friday*: 3 sets of 15 for the lower body.
> 6. *Saturday*: 5 sets of 5 reps for the upper body.
> 7. *Sunday*: 5 sets of 5 reps for the lower body.

The next question is always how often? You should do it (this month) three times a week. You can do all three days in a row if you prefer. My only suggestion is to not exercise the same muscles two days in a row. Your muscles need time to heal and recover. Generally this means, exercise a muscle group every other day. Eventually, you will want to do resistance training for each muscle group 3x/week. Performing strength-training 2x/week is generally considered maintenance.

> **Ex.** *Upper body →Monday and Wednesday*
> *Lower body →Tuesday*

Remember the theory of specificity and the SAID principle. If you lift heavy weights 3 sets of 10 for your biceps every other day, your biceps will get stronger—your back will not. I know it sounds simple, but it is amazing how many people think by working out there biceps and pecs, that their back and ankles would greatly improve. Again, this is why we want to develop a program that trains the whole body. We want your back to get just as much attention as your calf muscles.

By the end of the year, you will be performing resistance training more days of the week and it will be better balanced. For now, I suggest doing the weakest muscles two times per week and your stronger muscles only once.

Resistance training also benefits from variety and cross-training. If you do 3 sets of 10 biceps curls every other day with the same weight, your body gets very efficient at performing this act and will have to strain less and less to get it done, leaving you with less benefit from the exercise. Even something as simple as lowering the weight a little and doing 4 sets of 15 or raising the weight and doing 2 sets of 8 will present a different challenge for your body. If you do a lot of machine weights, try doing a few days or weeks here and there with the free weights.

Suspension bands are relatively new to the exercise world. I am going to take time here to talk about them because they are extremely space efficient with minimal cost ($50-120). They allow you to buy less equipment because you can do so much with them. They hang in any doorway. You can do hundreds of exercises for all body parts using a suspension band set. They use your body weight as resistance. There are upper/lower body exercises and trunk stability exercises. They can be used indoors or outside. My blog will have pictures and videos of various suspension band exercises. Another alternative is the kettle bell. These can be purchased with an instructional DVD for anywhere from $25-$100. Most of the exercises with a kettle bell involve repeated motion of major muscle groups and multiple parts of the body working together.

Obviously cost becomes an issue at this point (if it has not already). Do you need your own personal gym? Not necessarily. My equipment at home consists of three dumbbells, a soft mat, resistance tubing, and suspension bands—a whopping $120 in total. If you are creative, this is very doable and manageable on a tight budget. Hopefully this part was already completed in month 1 and you do not have to worry about it here.

The following table has a list of many exercises. The exercises at the top of each list are my "Best Bang For Your Buck" exercises. If you only have time for a few exercises, these are your go to moves (please remember that this is not an all-inclusive list).

| Upper Body | Trunk | Lower Body |
|---|---|---|
| Bicep Curls | Bridges | Squats |
| Triceps Pushes | Posterior-pelvic tilt | Lunges |
| Shoulder Abduction | Crunches | Heel raises |
| Shoulder External Rotation | Planks | Step-ups |
| Shoulder Internal Rotation | Heel Taps | Side lying hip abduction |
| Scapula Squeezes | Crunches with twist | |
| Chest Press | Crunch Bikes | |
| Serratus Punches | | |

The table below will be your resistance-training journal for at least the next month.

| Mon | Tues | Wed | Thurs | Fri | Sat | Sun |
|---|---|---|---|---|---|---|
| Legs (15min AM) Legs (15 min PM) | | Arms (20min AM) Arms (10min PM) | | | Arms (20min AM) Arms (10min PM) | |
| | | | | | | |
| | | | | | | |
| | | | | | | |

|  |  |  |  |  |  |  |
|--|--|--|--|--|--|--|
|  |  |  |  |  |  |  |
|  |  |  |  |  |  |  |
|  |  |  |  |  |  |  |
|  |  |  |  |  |  |  |
|  |  |  |  |  |  |  |

<u>Month 5 Checklist</u>
1. I have all the necessary equipment or gym membership to succeed ☐
2. I am performing resistance exercises for a total of 30 minutes 3 out of the 7 days in the week ☐
3. I have fit my resistance training comfortably into my existing schedule ☐

# Month 6: Flexibility

*Goal: By the end of the month you will perform 15 minutes of stretching and flexibility 2 out of 7 days in the week.*

Flexibility tends to be a tough sell. Most people do not see immediate results which make it hard to convince people they need to do it. During normal daily activities, most people will not notice limited flexibility. However, as you get older, flexibility becomes more and more important. As you get older, the elasticity of soft tissue in your body decreases (as water content decreases). It becomes harder and harder for people to perform simple tasks (getting in and out of bed, up and down stairs, in/out of a car). For this reason, it is important to start a flexibility regimen, even if it is only twice a week.

*What to Stretch*

I have found that the most important muscle group to stretch is the hamstrings. EVERYONE has tight hamstrings. I had a patient that came in complaining of low back pain for the past 4 months. His treatment was various stretches to improve hamstring flexibility—that's it! After 2 weeks, he was ready to move on with his life. The hamstrings attach around the back of the knee and up to your hips. If they are abnormally tight they can actually roll your hips down and backwards, putting extra strain on your back—a very common cause of low back pain. So if you stretch nothing else, stretch your hamstrings.

From my experience, you should also stretch your hips and trunk. Good flexibility in these muscles makes getting dressed, getting in/out of the car, etc. much easier as you get older. These are the most important, but a more complete routine will benefit you greatly.

*How to Stretch*

I have seen more variations of stretching than I have space to write about—everything from bouncing to just sitting there. Before any stretching you will want to perform a light warm-up just prior to stretching (something as simple as a 5 minute walk will be just fine!). To increase the length of your muscles (what I have been referring to as stretching), you want long hold times. My suggestion is 3 sets of 60-second holds (60 being the minimum). The longer you hold a muscle in a stretch position, the greater the stimulus you apply to the muscle to add links and lengthen. With longer holds you can also inhibit the nerve receptors that prevent your muscles from lengthening and relaxing. In other words, you make your nervous system relax and you can stretch more. If you have an extremely tight muscle, you should either do a light work out or put some heat on the muscles to help them relax before you start tugging on them.

Evidence does not support stretching before a work out to prevent injury. In fact, static stretching (3 sets, 60-second holds) has been shown to decrease the power a muscle can generate during sports and exercise immediately after stretching. There are contradicting reasons for this, but the bottom line is that stretching before exercise is not going to prevent any injuries. Think of your muscles as rubber bands. If you take a cold rubber band (your muscles before a work out) and start pulling on it, you run the risk of tearing it. On the other hand, if you lightly work with them and warm them up, when you pull, they stretch out much easier with less risk of snapping. The same holds true with our muscles. A more effective approach to prevent injuries is actually to perform a light warm-up (walking, biking, light exercise, etc.). That being said, after a workout seems to me like a great time to stretch. Your muscles will be loose and warmed up. This is a great time to sneak in a few stretches.

## How Often to Stretch

The answer varies widely depending on what you read and who you will talk to. What I tell all of my patients is—anytime you can, anytime you think about it. The following is my opinion based on what I have seen and read.

The answer will vary widely depending on your age and normal activity level. If you are younger (22 and younger) and are not in competitive sports, you probably do not have to worry much about stretching. A good, whole body routine twice a week will be sufficient (this is more than the majority of people do in most cases). If you are in a competitive sport in the younger age group, stretching more often (4 days a week) is advisable. This is especially true as you get deeper into the season and fatigue becomes a bigger issue and you start to tighten up.

In the middle aged group (22-45 year old), stretching 3 times a week should suffice. In this age group for the sedentary and/or leisure athlete, getting into a regular routine of stretching is good for maintaining normal flexibility.

In the older age group (45-older), I recommend at least some stretching every day. As you get older, your flexibility decreases. The reason why I suggest starting around 45 is that inflexibility creeps up on people and their activity becomes restricted before they know it. What I have noticed from most of my patients is that it sneaks up on you. I hear, "One day I was doing everything, and the next I could hardly look over my shoulder in the car" routinely. Flexibility is not something most people think about and it will catch up with you eventually. The older you get, the stiffer you get. At some point this will limit your ability to bend over and tie your shoes, get in and out of cars, move around in bed, etc. It becomes debilitating. Being proactive will help prevent the decline.

## Month 6 Checklist

1. I am stretching at least 15 minutes 2 out of 7 days during the week ☐

Half-Way There!

Congratulations. You are half-way through the program. Your life has changed drastically over the past 6-months (hopefully for the better). I hope you are starting to see positive changes in your health and are feeling better about exercise and being healthy. The next 6-months will be a challenge that I think you are ready for.

**Before moving on, let's assess what has happened.**

1. Planning Stage: You successfully set yourself up for a positive change. By the end of the month you had everything in place so that you could start your new life. ☐
2. You discovered what motivates you and organized a system of rewards and reinforcement. ☐
3. By the end of the third month you made the first meal of the day healthy and had healthy snacks during the day. ☐
4. By the end of the forth month you were performing 30 minutes of cardiovascular exercise 3 out of 7 days in the week. ☐
5. By the end of the fifth month you were performing 30 minutes of resistance exercise 3 out of 7 days in the week. ☐
6. By the end of the sixth month you were performing 15 minutes of stretching and flexibility 2 out of 7 days in the week. ☐

The table below shows what a normal week of yours should look like at this point.

| Mon | Tues | Wed | Thurs | Fri | Sat | Sun |
|---|---|---|---|---|---|---|
| Ate Healthy | Ate Healthy | Ate Healthy | Ate Healthy | Ate Healthy | Ate Healthy | Ate Healthy |
|  | Cardio-30min |  | Cardio-30min |  | Cardio-30min |  |
| Weight training 30min |  | Weight training 30min |  | Weight training 30min |  | Motivation: bought DVD ($8) |
|  |  | Stretched 15min |  |  |  | Stretched 15min |

## Half-Way Point

Age: _____     Height: _____     BMI: _____

Weight: _____     HR: _____     Body Fat %: _____

Blood Pressure: _____

Waist Size: _____     Are You Healthy? _____

What goals have you successfully met?
1. _____
2. _____
3. _____
4. _____
5. _____
6. _____
7. _____
8. _____
9. _____
10. _____

Are there any goals you would like to add?
1. _____
2. _____
3. _____
4. _____
5. _____

# Month 7: Planning/Maintenance

*Goal: Assess everything you have accomplished. Look for things that tripped you up or need to be changed/improved. Establish an updated plan of action.*

If you have successfully made it this far in the program, congratulations! Most people are unable to continue with a new lifestyle change this long. You should be very proud of your accomplishments and ready for the new challenges.

Now that you have completed the first round of challenges and goals, it is time to assess what has worked for you and what has not (please continue with your program during this month, this is not a time to drop everything!).

> If you have not already done so, get a journal/calendar/blog/computer program/or notebook of some kind to keep track of all your progress!

Here are just a few questions I came up with. They are regarding a number of problems friends, patients, and I have come across.

1. Is the gym too expensive? Is there a way to quit without being fined? Does the gym help motivate you to exercise still? Do you think you'd be better off getting your own equipment? Would working alone be easier for you?

2. Is your rewards system working? Are you looking forward to your rewards? Are you ready to make them less tangible (intrinsic)? If they are intrinsic, do you need the occasional tangible reward?

3. Are you enjoying the foods you are eating? Are they fulfilling your hunger cravings? Have you tried different recipes? Are you tired of your current diet? How often do you "cheat" on your current diet?

4. Are you enjoying your cardiovascular routine? Is it time to try something different? What are your options?

5. Are you enjoying your resistance training routine? Is it time to try something different? What are your options?

6. Are you enjoying your flexibility routine? Is it time to try something different?

7. Is it time for new sneakers/workout shoes (change running shoes about every 300 miles)? Is it time for new workout clothes?

8. Do you need a new play list to workout to? Have you tried working out with audiobooks to help pass the time? Do you prefer peace and quiet?

Now that you have looked at the past few months and have asked the necessary questions, it is time for you to fix things. In the coming months you are going to have to increase your time invested in this lifestyle change. Make sure that everything is arranged so that you can smoothly continue transitioning into your lifestyle transformation.

Month 7 Checklist

1. I have corrected any problems and am prepared to move on with my lifestyle change ☐

The following blank space is to give you space to jot some notes to yourself (things to do, preparations needed, phone numbers, etc).

Use this space for extra notes, phone numbers, goals, etc.

# Month 8: Motivation

*Goal: Start taking tangible rewards away. You do not want to need them! By the end of the month, you will be intrinsically rewarding yourself.*

  Finding something to motivate you is usually easier than this next step—taking it away. Just like a new puppy you are rewarding every time they use the bathroom outside and not on your bed, eventually you want to do these things without needing a reward. This new lifestyle needs to become just part of your routine. This is a very tricky part for most people. If you do not have something tangible to motivate you, why do it? It is another reason that internal gain is a great motivator, because you will always have that. My best friend loves the feeling he gets after a workout and actually looks forward to them daily. At the time I am writing this, I have been working out and eating healthy most days for the past 3 years. My drive at this point is purely internal. I know how important it is and I want to prolong my healthy years and quality of life for the rest of my life. Easier said than done. How do you do this, especially if your motivator is a "thing"?

  The first step is to cut back, not cut out. If you are rewarding yourself every week, make it every other week. The weeks you are not rewarding yourself with something, sit down on Sunday and make a list of reasons why you are making this change. It will serve as its own internal motivation.

Week 1:
Ex. So I can participate more with my children in sports.
1. _____
2. _____
3. _____
4. _____
5. _____

Week 2:
1. _____
2. _____
3. _____
4. _____
5. _____

    Are you proud of what you have accomplished and how it is helping you become a better, healthier person? You are doing something that most of the world cannot! You are changing for the better! 2/3 of the US population is overweight. 1/3 of the US population is obese. 1/3 of children are overweight (rising FAST). All of these numbers are rising. YOU are doing something positive to change these statistics. You are doing something to improve your quality of life.

    Each month, remove one "thing" reward and replace it with another list. This is a real list from a patient of mine. This is a sample of her Chapter 8.

Week 1: Went to a local concert.

Week 2:
1. __Improving my blood pressure _____
2. __Decreasing stress levels _____
3. __I am now able to go on walks in the neighborhood with my granddaughter. _____
4. ___I can garden all weekend without my knees hurting _____
5. ___Losing weight, slowly but surely _____

Week 3: Went to ice cream parlor

Week 4:
1. ___Feeling better about myself _____
2. ___Lowered my cholesterol _____
3. ___Fitting into smaller clothes _____
4. ___Spending more time in the lake with my grandkids _____
5. ___Rode a bike for the 1st time in 2 years _____

    The next month she had recorded 3 lists and 1 reward and so on. I realize it is easier said than done, but it can be done. Your turn!

Week 1: _____

Week 2:
1. _____
2. _____
3. _____
4. _____
5. _____

Week 3: _____

Week 4:
1. _____
2. _____
3. _____
4. _____
5. _____

Week 5: _____

Week 6:
1. _____
2. _____
3. _____
4. _____
5. _____

Week 7:
1. _____
2. _____
3. _____
4. _____
5. _____

Week 8:
1. _____
2. _____
3. _____
4. _____
5. _____

Week 9:
1. _____
2. _____
3. _____
4. _____
5. _____

Week 10:
1. _____
2. _____
3. _____
4. _____
5. _____

Week 11:
1. _____
2. _____
3. _____
4. _____
5. _____

Week 12:
1. _____
2. _____
3. _____
4. _____

5. _____

      I know you might be thinking that there are a lot of lists and you will not be able to come up with that many different things to internally motivate you. I think it will be easier than you think. Remember, it does not have to be different things every week. If losing cholesterol is still driving you, write it down! A suggestion with the cholesterol (and weight, blood levels, etc.), make it a challenge. Obviously you want to get the numbers into safe ranges, but set a realistic number for yourself and aim for it the next time you get blood drawn. I have even had patients (husband and wife) competing to see who can lower their cholesterol by the greatest amount safely.

<u>Month 8 Checklist</u>

1. I am only rewarding myself intrinsically ☐

# **Month 9: Diet**

*Goal: Have a healthy lunch and dinner 6 out of 7 days in the week.*

The last time we visited your diet, the goal was to have a healthy breakfast and snacks. This time we are just upping the ante to include lunch and dinner. This is tough and will take some working in to. At this point you are already eating a healthy breakfast and snacks 7 days of the week. Lunch and dinner are a little harder. Hopefully by now, you are starting to venture into the world of healthier foods and are developing a taste for some new things.

Like all the other steps, start small. If you are not eating a single healthy lunch and/or dinner any night of the week, start by eating 2 healthy lunches and 2 healthy dinners each week. They can be on the same or different days. Like the exercise, I would suggest spreading them out so you are doing multiple meals (breakfast + lunch/dinner) each day rather than many healthy meals only a couple days of the week. Start paying even more attention to nutrition labels. Look for things high in fiber and vitamins and low in cholesterol and calories.

Sandwiches are easy lunches that you can make very healthy. Just remember that deli meats are loaded with salt! Bring a couple healthy sides to make sure you are full at the end of the meal (granola/blueberries and yogurt is my personal favorite).

Dinner is the real catch. By the time you get home, exercise, relax, deal with everything else going on in your life, the idea of cooking yourself a healthy dinner has long since left your head. What do you do? Fortunately, there are dozens of cookbooks with recipes that can be made healthily and in a small time frame. These are phenomenal and you should really look into a couple. Most will also include a nutrition chart which helps immensely.

One of the best tips I can offer you is to plan ahead. This applies for all meals and snacks, but especially dinner. An easy thing I like to do is cook too much dinner and have leftovers for a day or two for lunch. Another option is to grill/cook/etc a few breasts of chicken (or other meats) and then freeze them. For a few nights afterwards you will easily be able to pull out your frozen (already cooked) chicken, the frozen bag of veggies (frozen veggies have been shown to have more vitamins and nutrients than fresh fruits/veggies that can be lost trying to preserve them for supermarket shelves), and a healthy, complete dinner can be ready in mere seconds. If you see the "pre-prepared" meals in the supermarket—BEWARE. These tend to be packed with more salt and fat than you could ever imagine. Cook and freeze it yourself!

Lunch can be done similarly. Pack it the night before (right before bed) so you can just grab it as you walk out the door in the morning. Then you do not have to get up any earlier to pack your lunch in the morning (same is true for snacks).

If one of your goals is to get more fruits and veggies in a day, create supplies. Most fruits and veggies take a little prep (cleaning, cutting, etc). If you are planning on having cucumbers and carrots as a snack tomorrow, clean and cut a couple days worth tonight.

For all of these meals and snacks, you need to find some storage containers. I put my meals and snacks in a couple of these every night. This is a good way to watch your portion control and a good way to watch your progress (made 5 containers every day in the start, now its only 3), or lack there of. This only makes it easier for you. If you spend a few minutes extra Sunday night preparing all of these ready to eat meals for the week, things go a lot more smoothly and you feel like you are wasting less time during the week worrying about food. If you are trying to save money, this is much cheaper than eating out, even at cheaper restaurants.

The last thing I'll say is—do not prepare hungry. If you are sitting in front of your fridge at 9:30PM Sunday night trying to think of what to make for the weeks meals and you are starving, you will prepare way too much. You will over-pack for the week. Just like people say, do not go to the supermarket hungry, do not prepare your meals hungry. You will over-pack and over-eat.

*A Few Sample Days*

| Day 1 | Breakfast: cereal, banana, water<br>Lunch: PB & J, yogurt with granola, orange juice<br>Dinner: grilled chicken, broccoli, corn, glass of wine<br>Snacks: grapes, carrots, cucumbers, wheat crackers |
|---|---|
| Day 2 | Breakfast: toast, grapefruit, water<br>Lunch: grilled chicken salad, wheat crackers<br>Dinner: grilled fish with lemon, mashed potatoes, side salad, water<br>Snacks: yogurt, tomato and basil |
| Day 3 | Breakfast: scrambled eggs, toast, orange, coffee<br>Lunch: grilled chicken sandwich, side salad<br>Dinner: pasta salad, apple, water<br>Snacks: carrots, watermelon |
| Day 4 | Breakfast: cereal with banana, apple, water<br>Lunch: Ham and cheese sandwich, salad, juice<br>Dinner: Tomato with mozzarella and basil, fruit salad<br>Snacks: granola bar, yogurt, orange, celery |

Month 9 Checklist

1. I am eating healthy lunch and dinners 6 out of 7 days a week ☐

# Month 10: Cardio

*Goal: 30 minutes per day, every day. Develop a cardio routine.*

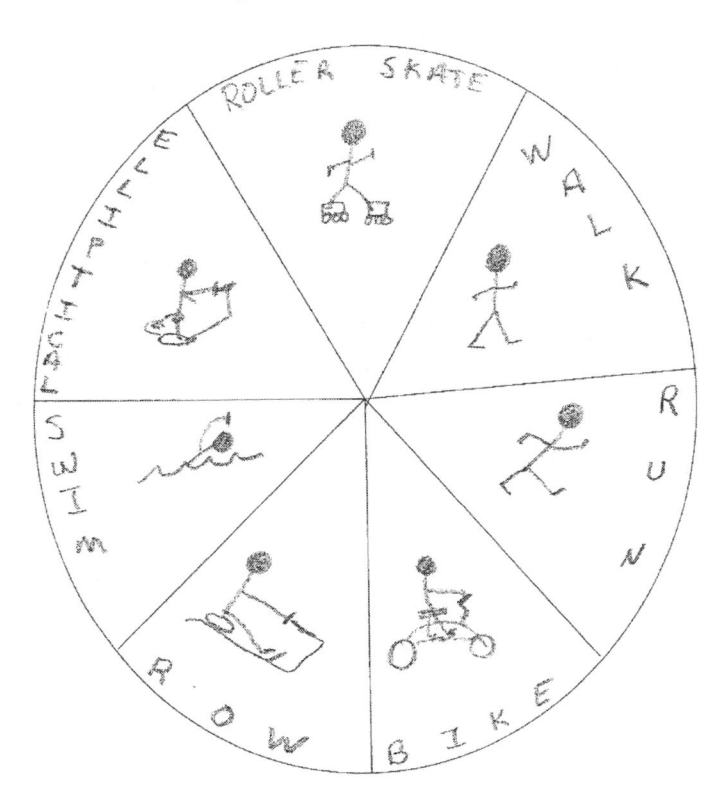

The goals are getting tougher. This time you are not only upping your daily dose of cardio, but you are also learning to plan your workouts ahead. This does not have to be anything complicated or convoluted. Keep it simple. So many people want to be professional athletes and come up with these insanely specific workouts.

*Ex. 20 min bike at 75% VO$_2$Max, 5 min at 90%, 5 min at 50%.*

You will spend ¾ of the time checking your pulse and figuring out needless equations. Unless you are training and trying to get every last ounce of benefit in order to improve performance by minuscule numbers, then just do something challenging.

My example for you:
20 min bike at intensity to get you breathing moderately well
5 min of biking at top speed
5 min of very light biking to relax
End of work out—feel tired, heart rate is up, sweating

Yes, training in target heart rate zones and monitoring your % of VO$_2$Max (the amount of oxygen you can use) is important for performance based training and can be useful for health based training, but is certainly not necessary. I think the *tired rule* works just fine. If, at the end of the work out you are really tired, then you have probably done enough to get some benefit out of it. If you get to the end of the workout and feel that you could go on for 3 more hours, your workout has not been hard enough and you need to increase the intensity next time.

*Reminders on How to Workout*

A suggestion about "How" to perform your cardio is to keep it variable. Keep it variable in the workout and between workouts. In the workout, go hard for 5 minutes, tone it down for 5 minutes, ramp it up to a moderate intensity, then bring it back down. It forces your body to constantly adapt and adjust to changing needs (similar to real life). A lot of the new research I have been reading is showing very positive effects of interval training. Between workouts change it up. On Monday bike for 30 minutes at a constant/moderate rate. When you bike again on Wednesday, sprint the first 10 seconds of every minute, then relax for 50 seconds. In addition to challenging your body, it also helps change up the workouts over time (they can get monotonous real quick if you ,are not careful). Remember there are many ways to get your cardio exercise in.

The last "How" topic before jumping into how to organize your schedule is overload. It is one of the most common principles in exercise prescription and can be applied to all types of exercise. As explained earlier, it means you have to continuously make things more difficult. For example, if you use the sprinting the first 10 seconds of every minute example, after you have done this a while, it will get easier and easier until you are not getting significant benefits workout anymore. If you continue to stay at that level, you will never improve, only maintain. To make this harder try sprinting 15 seconds or upping the intensity of the 50 second slow time. Always make your work out harder and more challenging if you want to continue to improve.

*Reminder on Organization*

So how do we fit this in to our crazy schedule? An important rule to remember is that the ACSM and AHA both state that you need 30 minutes of moderate physical activity every day. The important part of this rule is that you can do 10 or 15 minutes at a time which makes squeezing it into your day easier. Go for a quick jog before your morning shower and a quick jog right after you get home. If you are fortunate enough to have a good lunch break, and even equipment at your disposal, work out at lunch! Other people need to get it all done in one shot. My personal preference is running in the morning before I have the whole day to convince myself I do not really have to do it after work. For right now, try and get in to a normal routine. Once you have established a routine and start getting bored with it, this is when you should think about changing it up.

Many people will start as, and even become, a weekend-warrior. These are the people that do nothing active all week and then try and do a week's worth of exercise in 2 days. I will save you the trouble and tell you it does NOT work. A lot of people get injured doing this because they over-train past fatigue on these days. Muscle strains and pains are common with these types of workouts. A better idea is to do something every day to build strength and endurance.

*A usual day for me*

*Run before work*
*Weights over lunch*
*Stretching/core training after work.*

It works best for me to split everything up. I have also found that working out in the middle of the workday really splits things up nicely and gives me a little boost for the afternoon.

When are your favorite times to do cardio?
1. _____
2. _____
3. _____
4. _____
5. _____

When are some realistic times for you to fit it in?
1. _____
2. _____
3. _____
4. _____
5. _____

What are some ways you can vary your workouts?
1. _____
2. _____
3. _____
4. _____
5. _____

**Here is a Cardio table. Fill in your daily activities. Fill in the activity and the amount of time.**

| Mon | Tues | Wed | Thurs | Fri | Sat | Sun |
|---|---|---|---|---|---|---|
| Bike (35) | Run (20) | Run (25) | Bike (30) | Walk (60) | Row (40) | Walk (60) |
|  |  |  |  |  |  |  |
|  |  |  |  |  |  |  |
|  |  |  |  |  |  |  |
|  |  |  |  |  |  |  |
|  |  |  |  |  |  |  |
|  |  |  |  |  |  |  |
|  |  |  |  |  |  |  |
|  |  |  |  |  |  |  |
|  |  |  |  |  |  |  |
|  |  |  |  |  |  |  |
|  |  |  |  |  |  |  |

I mentioned VO$_2$Max earlier. As the intensity of your exercise goes up, so does the amount of oxygen you take in. At some point you reach a maximum where you can work out harder and harder, but the amount of oxygen you take in and use will not increase. This signifies the maximum amount of oxygen your body can take in to be used.

Why is this important? For those of you who are concerned about exercising in a target heart rate zone, knowing your VO$_2$Max can be very useful. A target heart rate zone is a range of your heart rate or VO$_2$Max that you try and work out in. It is an objective way of gauging how hard you are working out.

The easiest way is to use your heart rate. A safe way to use your heart rate as a gauge is with the Karvonen formula:

**Target Heart Rate = ((max HR − resting HR) × %Intensity) + resting HR**

You will use this equation twice, once for the lower end of intensity and once for the upper end. The intensity in which you choose to work out is totally up to you. Anywhere from 60-80% is a good average zone.

The other option is to exercise based on a percentage of your $VO_2Max$. This requires far more knowledge and usually some equipment to make it more accurate—way above what is needed for the people reading this book.

Month 10 Checklist

1. I am performing at least 30 minutes of cardio every day ☐

2. I enjoy the type of cardio exercise I am currently doing ☐

# Month 11: Resistance

*Goal: By the end of the month you will do resistance training at least 30 minutes per day, every day of the week.*

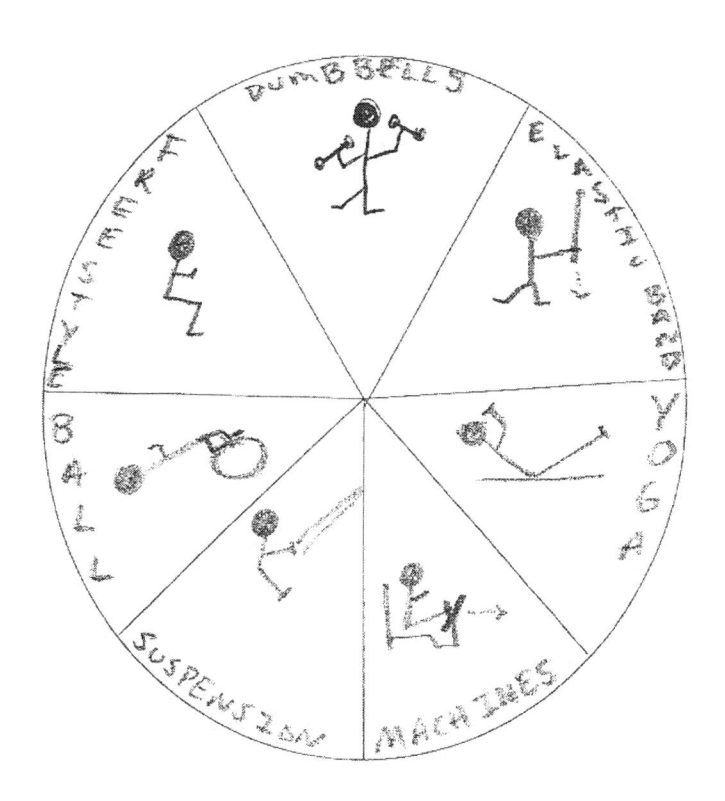

111

We have already discussed the role of the muscles and nerves in building your strength and the many other health benefits. This chapter is aimed at improving your resistance training routine and extending it to 7 days per week. We want to add variety to your workout to improve it and keep it interesting.

The last time we discussed resistance training was in the 5th month of your transformation. At this point you are performing resistance training 3 times per week for a total of 30 minutes each of those days. Most people at this point have a normal routine they follow (Tuesday/Thursday→Arms, Saturday→Core/legs. All with machines). The pie chart from the previous page is just to remind you that there are many ways of getting the necessary resistance training. If you are bored with your current routine, now is the time to start introducing new activities gradually.

> This week you should try and do 5 days of resistance training. Try 3 days with your normal routine and change it up for the 4th and 5th days in the week. OR Normal routine/change/normal routine/change/normal routine.

Sometimes, there are constraints on how much variation there can be because of time, money, etc. Within each type of training, there are different ways to perform activities.

One way is to change the pace. This can be used with elastic bands, suspension system, dumbbells, machines, and freestyle! Most people perform 3 sets of 10 reps at the same pace, for every exercise, every time. The down side is that your body gets very efficient at this type of work and it becomes less of a challenge for the working muscles. Try the same exercises, but in one direction slow down significantly. Take the bicep curls. Curl up the weight at the same pace you always have. Now on the way down, go reaaaallllyyyy slow. Do this for every repetition. Warning—you might be a little sore and tired the next day. At the gym, people refer to these as "negatives" or "eccentrics". Whatever you call them, they are a great way to build muscle once you have built a good foundation of strength (as you already have after month 5!).

Plyometrics are a different form of resistance training that involves explosive movements.

> These are only to be performed by people with a solid base of strength and are not for everyone. If you know a physical therapist, strength and conditioning specialist, or trainer, it would be advisable to consult with them to make sure you are prepared for plyometric training.

Plyometric exercises involve a quick stretch to the muscle and an immediate full force contraction (called the stretch-shortening cycle). This type of exercise increases the nervous system involvement and recruits more motor units in the muscle to create a stronger contraction in the muscle. Most of these exercises involve some kind of jumping motion. The number of repetitions/session varies among sources. Most recommendations I have seen for novices state 80 contractions/session, with up to 150 contractions/session for advanced athletes. My suggestion is to start very slow. These are very difficult and hard on your body. I tell people to start with 10. Wait 2 days and see how those muscles feel. If your muscles are still sore, stick with 10 until the pain stops after workouts. Once you can do 10 without any symptoms a couple days later, bump it to 20 and so on. Plyometrics can be performed by all ages if done correctly. My suggestion is to get some professional guidance to learn how to properly perform these exercises.

Who are some professionals in your area that could help you?
1. _____ Phone # _____
2. _____ Phone # _____
3. _____ Phone # _____
4. _____ Phone # _____
5. _____ Phone # _____

Most people think Olympic lifting is only for the seasoned veteran. To do it like the professionals, this is true. But most of us are not professionals and we still want different ways to get stronger. Olympic lifting is basically two movements: the snatch and the clean-and-jerk. The snatch is where the exerciser lifts the bar from the ground straight overhead in one fluid motion landing in the squat position. The clean is where the bar is picked up from the ground onto the person's shoulders. The jerk is where the bar is lifted overhead and the person ends in the lunge position (one foot bent in front of the other). Both motions require full-body participation and are therefore fantastic exercises to perform. My suggestion is to seek professional help initially to focus solely on form. You want to be able to perform both of these movements holding an un-weighted bar with perfect form before ever thinking about adding weights. Be careful, most trainers want to add weight right away. Trust me, become a perfectionist about form. When you have done that, start adding weight and you will reap the benefits.

Suspension bands are a new variation in the exercise world. They take advantage of your body weight for resistance. The anchor is hung over a door or in a tree and you hold on to handles at the end of 2 bands. Upper body, core, and lower body exercises can be performed with these bands. Where and/or how you decide to stand will affect the resistance you will work against. These are an easy way for beginners to get started. For $50 you can get a set of bands and a small instructional booklet to help get you started (deluxe versions start around $100) without any other equipment. They really are a great deal and are a great way to vary your exercise program.

Kettle bells are the new craze. They are essentially medicine balls with a handle. Anyone can perform simple kettle bell exercises. The most important thing to do is to perform these activities with proper form. Most of the movements require a swinging motion that requires all of your trunk muscles to be activated to maintain stability through the whole motion. If done correctly, these are great whole body workouts.

What are some exercises out there that you have not tried?
1. _____
2. _____
3. _____
4. _____
5. _____

What are some exercises out there that you want to try?
1. _____
2. _____
3. _____

**Fill out the table below throughout this month.**

| Date | Total Time | Activity | Feelings |
|---|---|---|---|
| 4-30-11 | 45 (all AM) | Suspension bands | Great change of pace |
| 5-2-11 | 30 (AM/PM) | Olympic lifting | Too intense for me |
|  |  |  |  |
|  |  |  |  |
|  |  |  |  |
|  |  |  |  |
|  |  |  |  |
|  |  |  |  |
|  |  |  |  |
|  |  |  |  |

## Month 11 Checklist

1. I am performing at least 30 minutes of resistance training every day ☐

2. I enjoy the type of resistance training I am currently doing ☐

# Month 12: Wrapping it Up

*Goal: Assess what you have done so far, look for potential pitfalls, adjust routines, etc.*

It is time to wrap your journey up. Over the next month you will need to finalize your workout routine and secure the continuation of your new lifestyle. We have a few major categories: Planning, Motivation, Diet, Cardio, Resistance, and Flexibility.

Your planning has been a significant portion of your journey as the major topic in 2 full months and a large part of this chapter. It is such a crucial part of the lifestyle improvement and is always ignored (which is why I have drawn so much attention to it!). At this point, you should be a member of a gym and/or have the necessary equipment to perform activities at home. You should have a calendar to help organize all of these new additions and activities. Your exercise and diet should fit smoothly/seamlessly into your new life.

Motivation goes right along with planning as underappreciated when developing a healthy lifestyle change (or poorly organized, set up for failure). Use something that works for you. Remember to change it up if your current form of motivation is not working for you. Be proud of what you have accomplished. Be excited about your potential for further improvement.

Healthy diet can transform your life. It can affect your energy levels, make you feel good, help you lose weight, and become healthier (among so many other benefits). We have talked a lot about your diet and some specifics about why you choose certain foods and not others. At this point in the program, you should be eating healthy all the time. Remember though, it is OK to splurge occasionally. Research shows that it is good for you mentally and behaviorally to eat differently sometimes. Going out to eat at a restaurant twice in a month is great! Eat, drink, and be merry. The problem starts when this becomes a staple of your normal diet. Eat in moderation. Eat a varied and colorful diet.

Cardiovascular exercise might be the single most important thing you can do for yourself. It does not tend to be a fan favorite, but it could not be more important to your health and longevity. Performing daily cardiovascular exercise will transform your life for the better.

Resistance training is usually peoples' "go-to move" when beginning exercise. This is partially because no one likes cardio and partially because everyone thinks they can just lift a few weights and create a smokin' bod. Remember to be creative with your routine. If you get done with a workout and you are not tired and thought it was easy, so did your body. You need to make it harder—increase the weight/reps or even the activities you are doing. Always challenge your body to adapt. Always challenge your body to do more.

We have covered every topic you need to succeed in this lifestyle change. As you come to the last few pages of this book, what are some areas that you feel need some fine tuning this last month?

1. _____
2. _____
3. _____
4. _____
5. _____

Before making any new changes to your program, address these. These small problems can become a hassle. This program should run smoothly and efficiently.

Once you have addressed these, start thinking about new goals for yourself. At this point in the program, you want to make long term goals for yourself. Where do you want to be in 6, 12, 24 months? What are some things you can work towards? In 12 months, would you like to run a marathon? Finish a triathlon?

What are some long-term goals?
1. _____
2. _____
3. _____
4. _____
5. _____

Month 12 Checklist

1. I have proper workout clothing/shoes for all activities I will be performing…☐
2. I have a gym membership or all of the necessary equipment to carry out my daily activity routine…☐
3. I have a safe place at home or to go to exercise…☐
4. I have a local supermarket(s) that carry the foods I will need to maintain a healthy and varied diet…☐
5. I have a system in place to make sure I will eat healthily every day…☐
6. I have allotted time in my daily life to allow for at least 30 minutes of resistance training, 30 minutes of cardiovascular training, and flexibility on the required days…☐
7. I have a large calendar to help organize my day around getting healthy…☐
8. I have a journal to record my diet and exercise for each day…☐

**Insert a picture of yourself.**

## **INDEX OF EXERCISES**

\*\*\* This is by no means an all-inclusive collection of exercises. These are included to show you good/safe exercises for you to incorporate into your routine.\*\*\*

## Bicep Curls

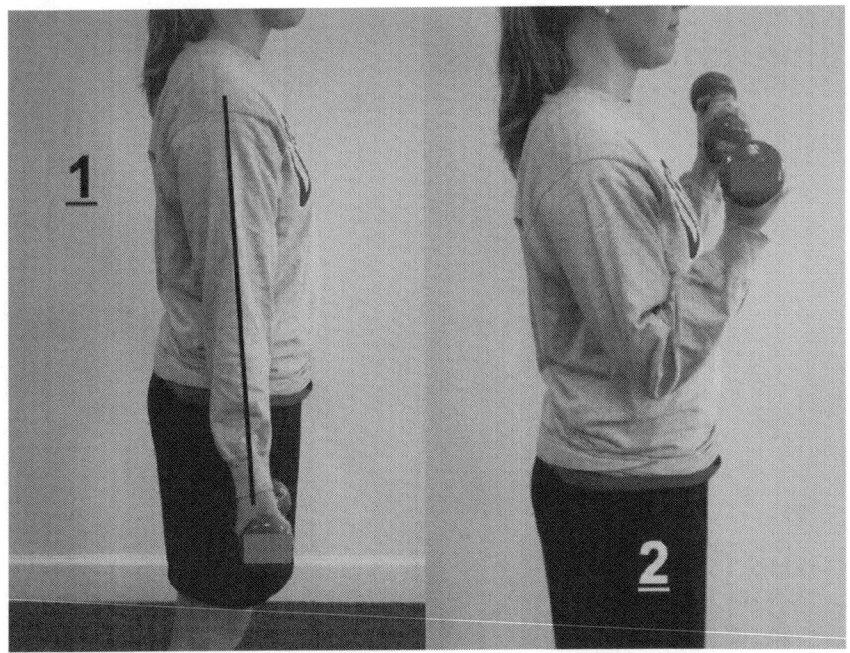

How to: Start with arms shoulder width apart and palms facing forward. Bend only at your elbow. Your shoulders should not move. Make sure to breath out on the way up and breath in as you let the weights slowly back down.

Variations: You can perform this with your palms starting facing forward, in towards your hips, or facing backwards.

## Bike Twists

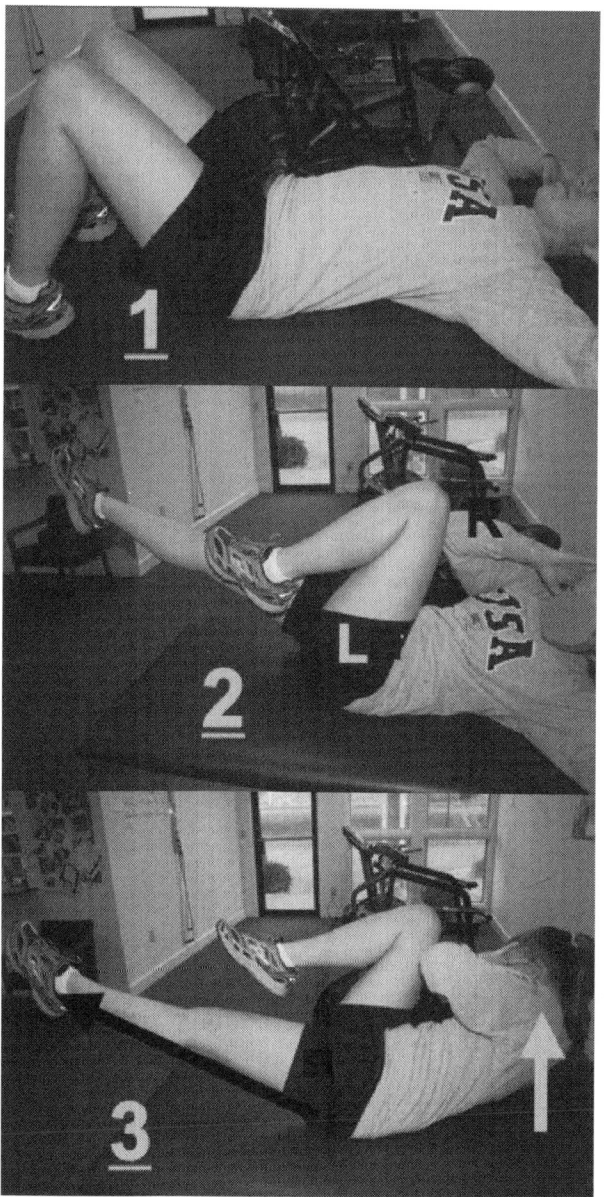

How To: Start by bringing both knees off the mat and curling your trunk up with your abs. Next, bring your right elbow and touch it to your left knee. Without going back to the starting position, twist and bring your left elbow to your right knee and repeat! This is an advanced move; please make sure you have sufficient strength and motion before performing this.

## Bridges

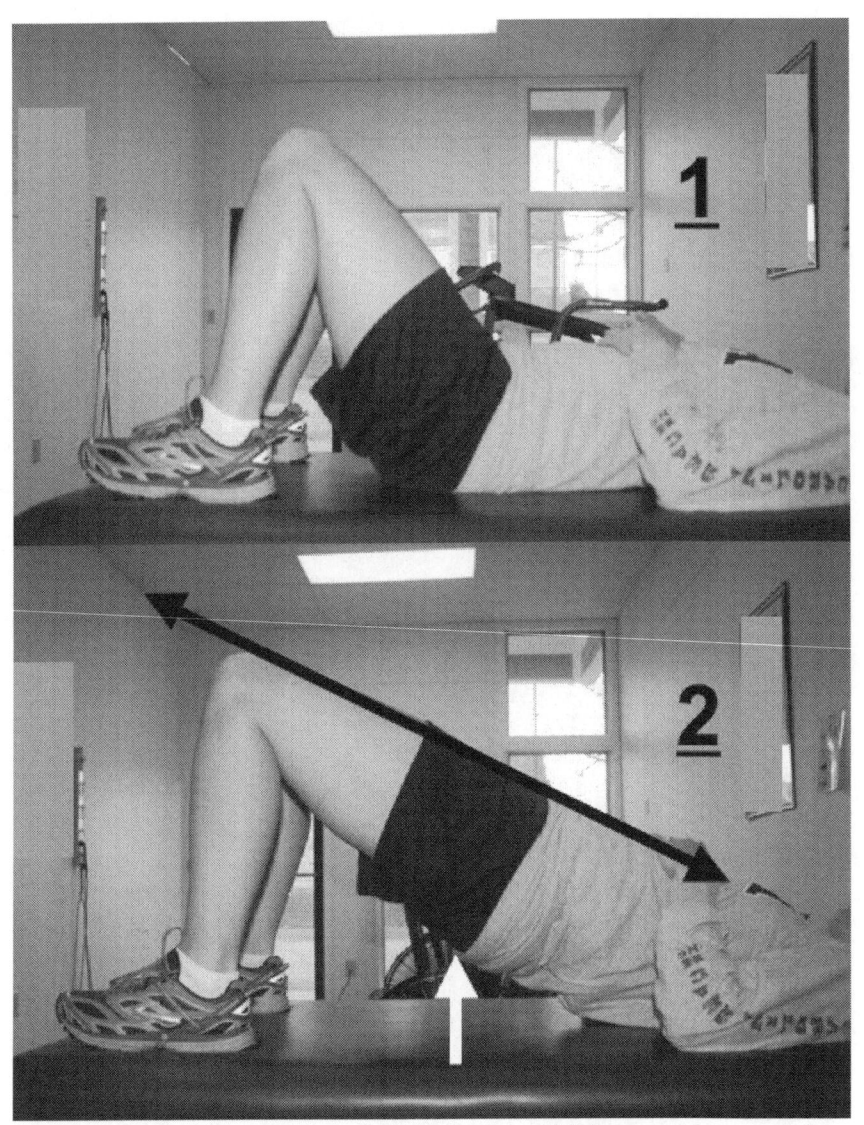

How to: From the starting position, you will lift your hips straight up towards the ceiling. You may push down through your feet, squeeze your gluteal muscles (buttocks), and contract your low back muscles. Be mindful not to arch your back. You want to end with a straight line from your knees to your shoulders.

## Chest Press

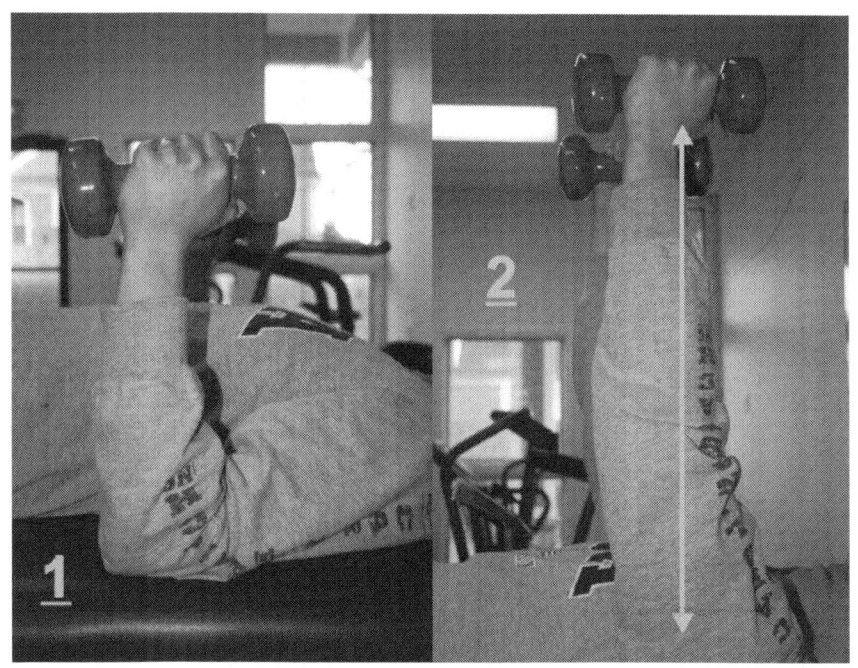

How to: Start with your elbows bent and resting on the floor/surface. Push the weights straight up into the air and fully extend/straighten your elbows.

Variations: You can push starting with your palms facing together (pictured) or with your palms facing your feet.

## Crunch

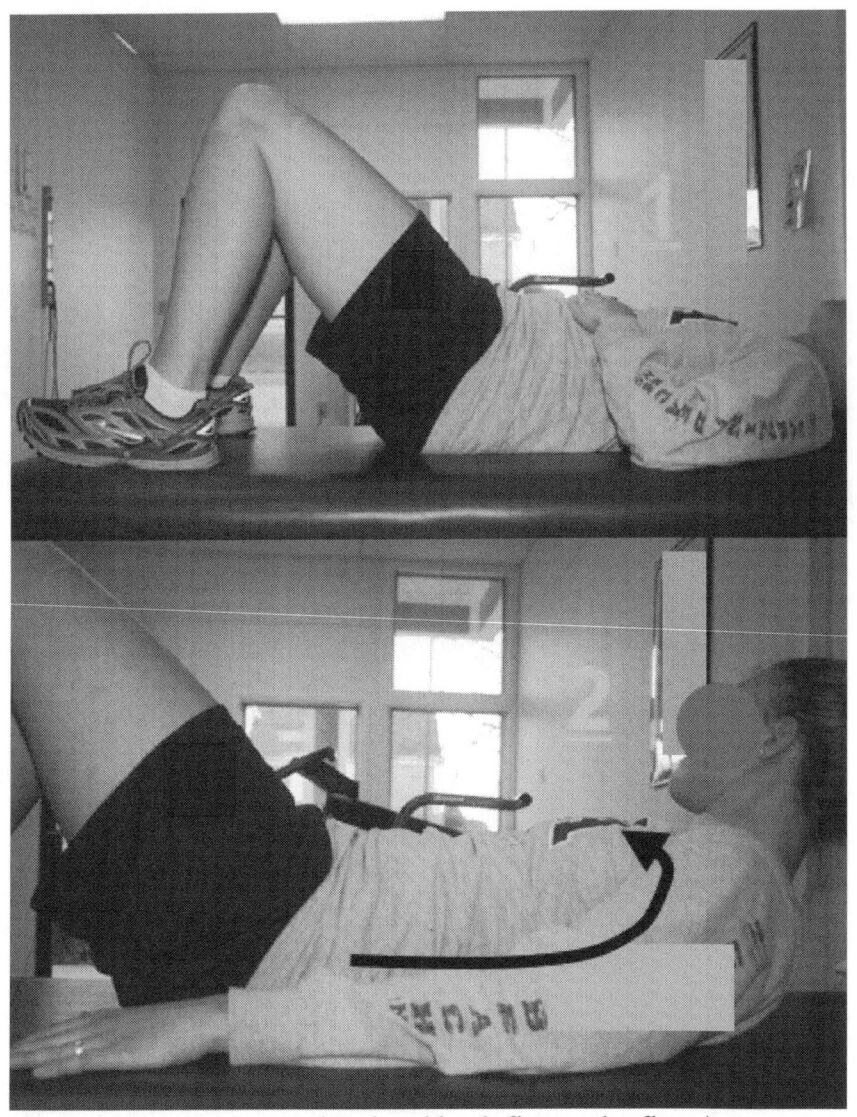

How to: Start with your head and back flat on the floor/mat. Contract your abdominal muscles and slowly raise your upper trunk off the mat. One way to make sure you do this correctly is to have your hands flat on the mat (pictured) and reach towards your feet on both sides with your hands flat on the mat at all times.

## Crunch With Twist

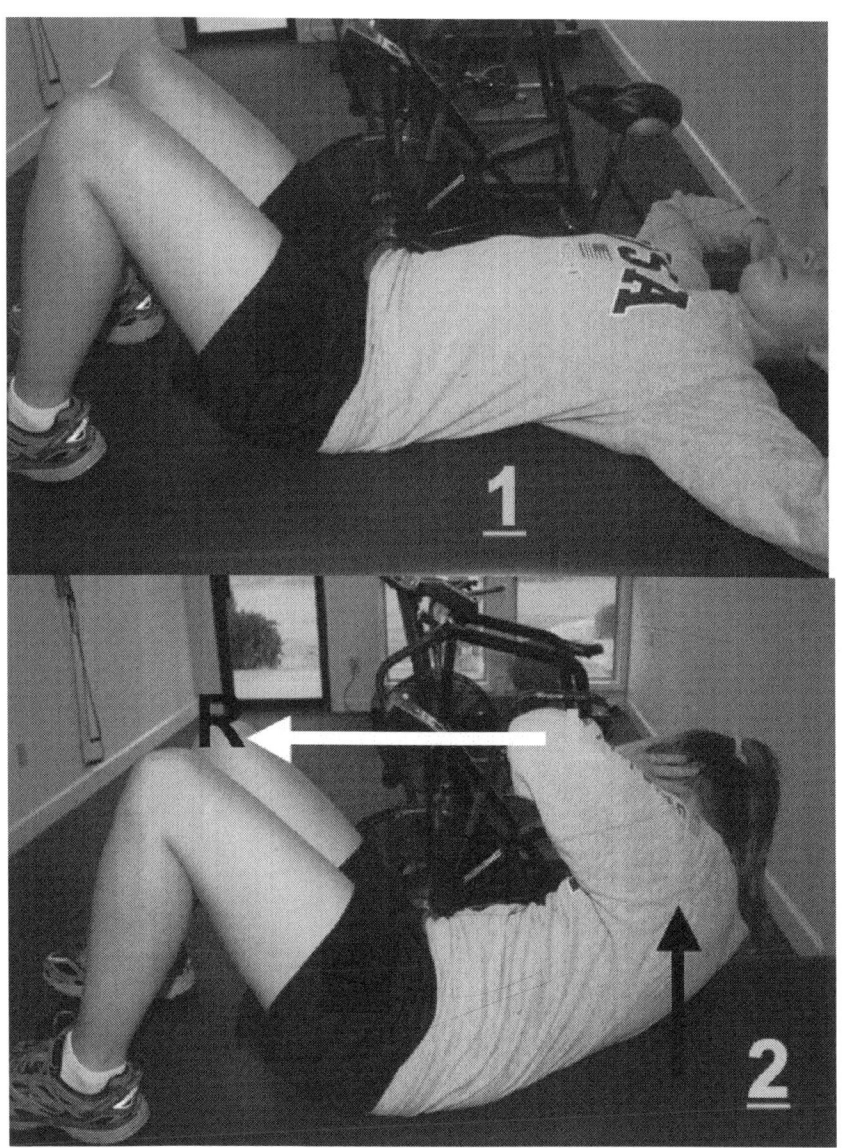

How to: Start with your head and back flat on the floor/mat. Contract your abdominal muscles and slowly raise your upper trunk off the mat. As you reach the top, slowly twist your left elbow towards your right knee. Then, slowly return to the starting position and repeat with a twist in the opposite direction.

## Heel Raise

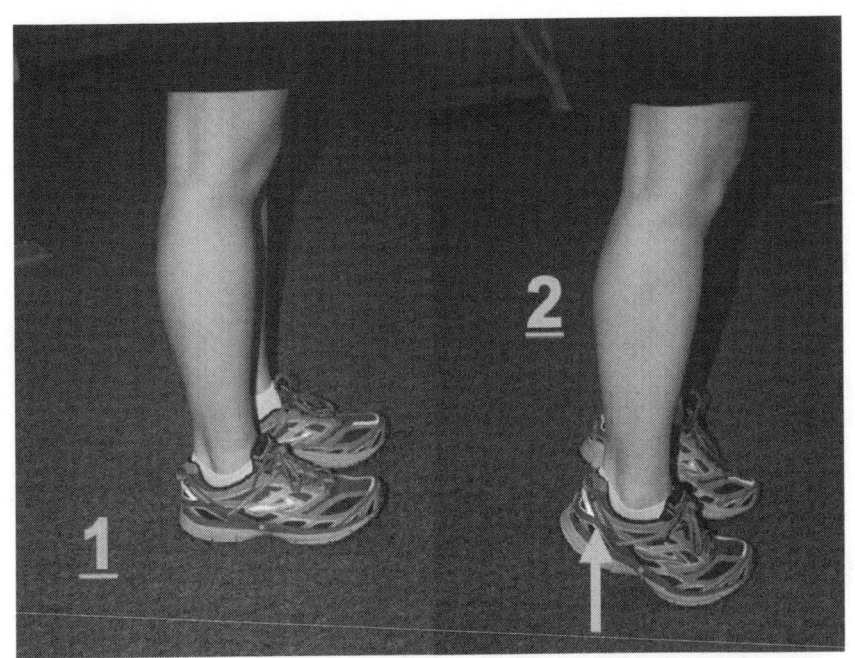

How to: Start with your feet flat on the floor. Push up on to your toes using only your calves. A common mistake is to swing your hips and knees forward for the momentum to get on your toes. Some people even try a mini-hop. To gain maximal benefit, try to generate all of the force from your calves without extra help.

Variations: To make this easier, you can do it in the seated position. This targets a slightly different muscle group, but is a good place to start. Another way to vary this is to use only one leg (make sure you have something to hold to balance on).

## Heel Taps

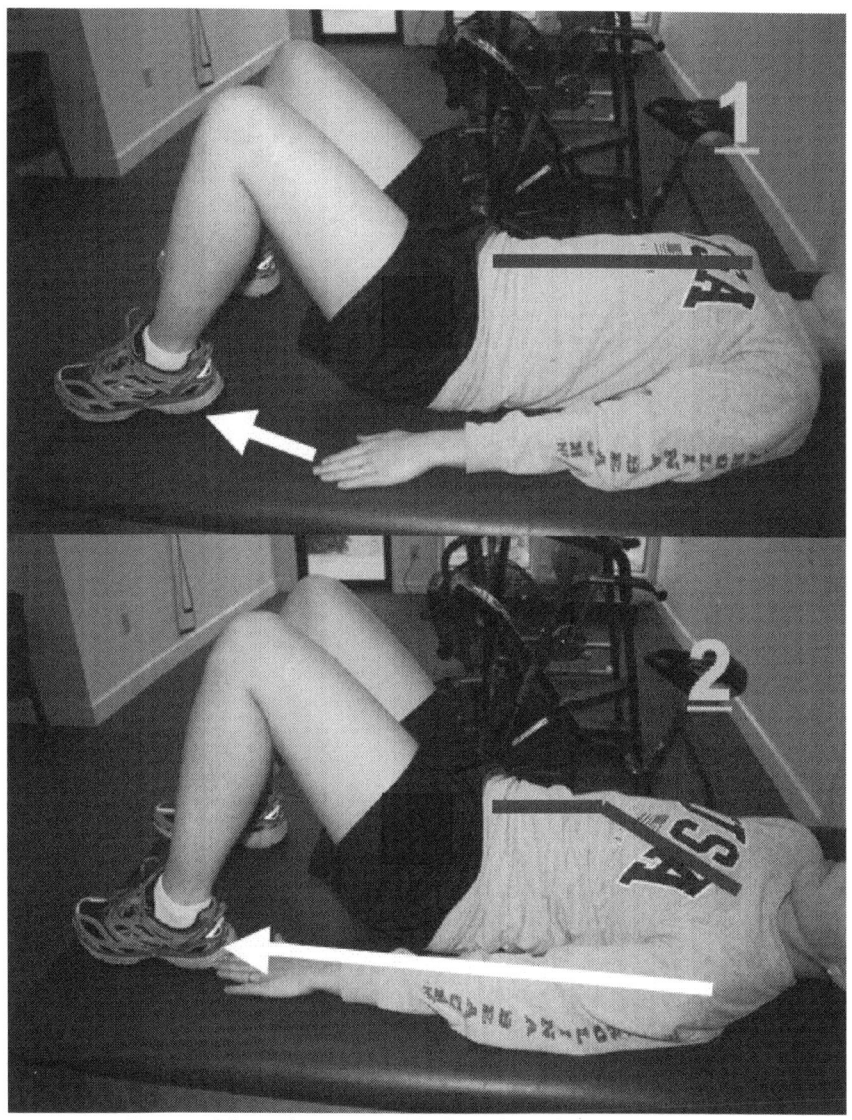

How to: Start with a short crunch (head and upper back off the mat with abs contracted). Next tilt and reach for your left heel and then swing to the right heel without returning to the starting position.

## Lunges

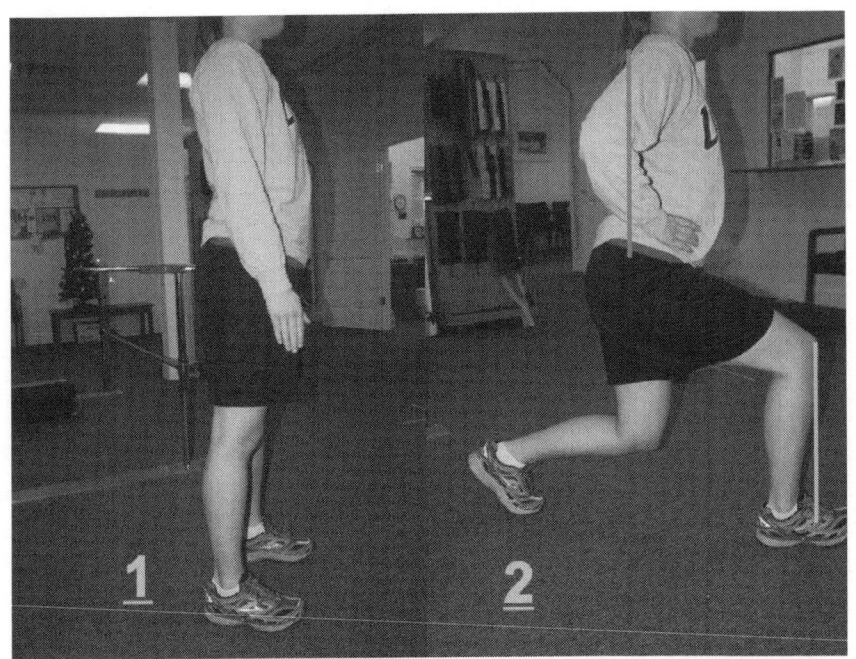

How to: Start with feet shoulder width apart. Step out with your right foot and bend both the left and right knee. Make sure that your forward knee (the one bearing most of the weight) does not progress over your toes (as shown by vertical green line). Keep your back straight through the entire process (orange line). Then step back to the starting position and step out with your left leg.

## Planks

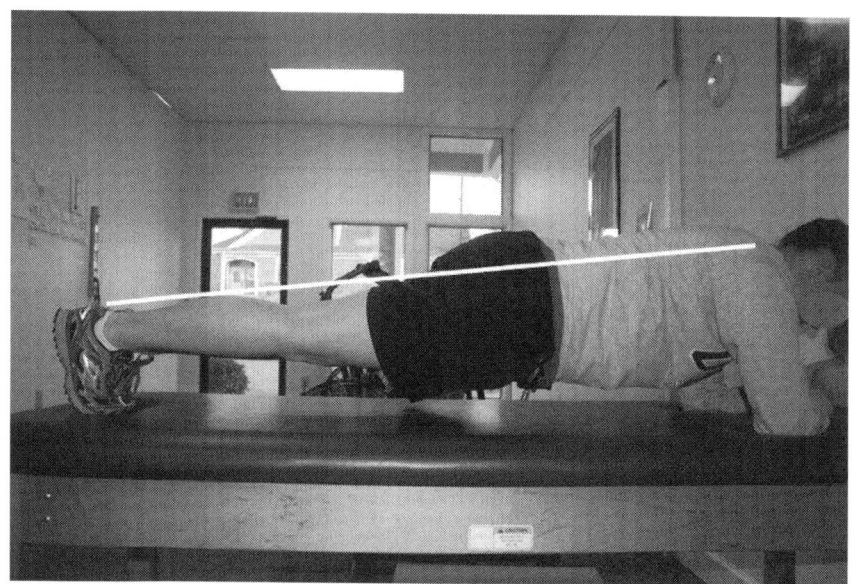

How to: Hold the position pictured above. Maintain your legs, hips, and back in a perfectly straight line. When it becomes difficult to hold and your form starts to falter, relax and take a breather.

## Posterior Pelvic Tilt

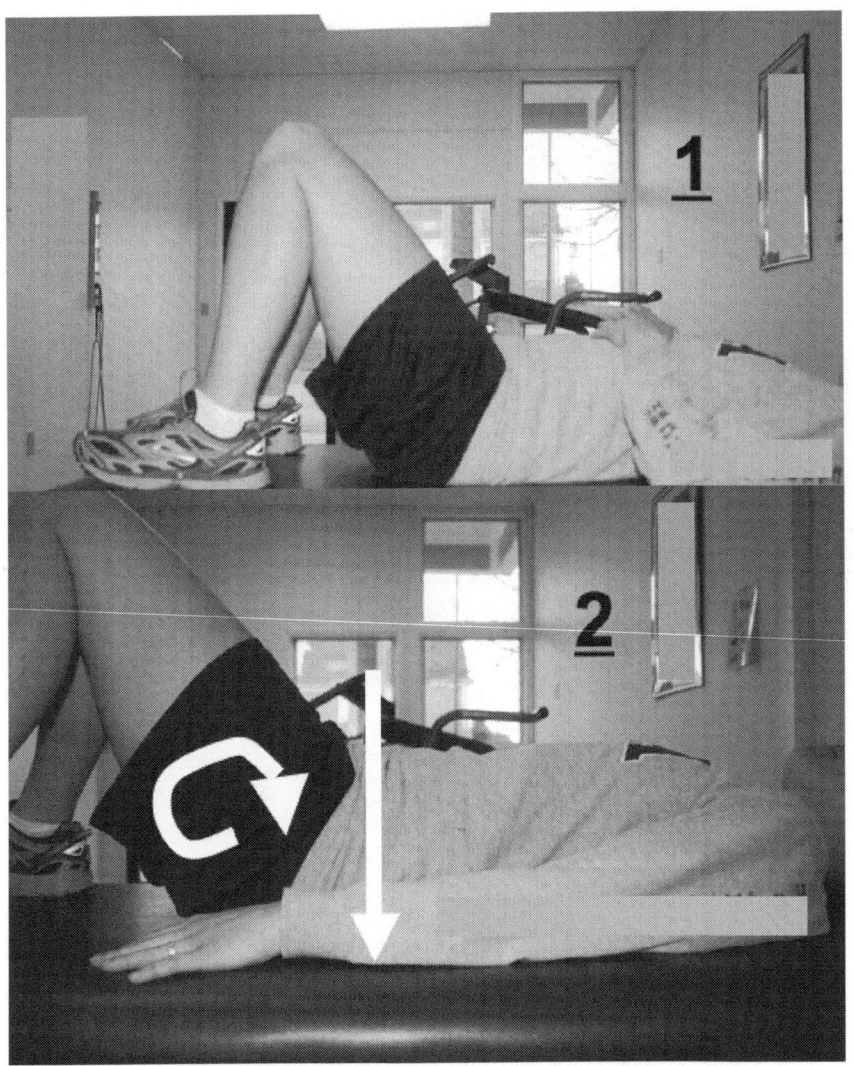

How to: For this exercise you are rolling your hips backwards, contracting your abs, and pushing your low back down into the bed/mat/floor. If you are arching your back, you are doing it wrong. If you are pushing through your feet, you are doing it wrong. If you are having trouble, place a small object in the small of your back and try to push it down into the table.

Scapular Squeezes

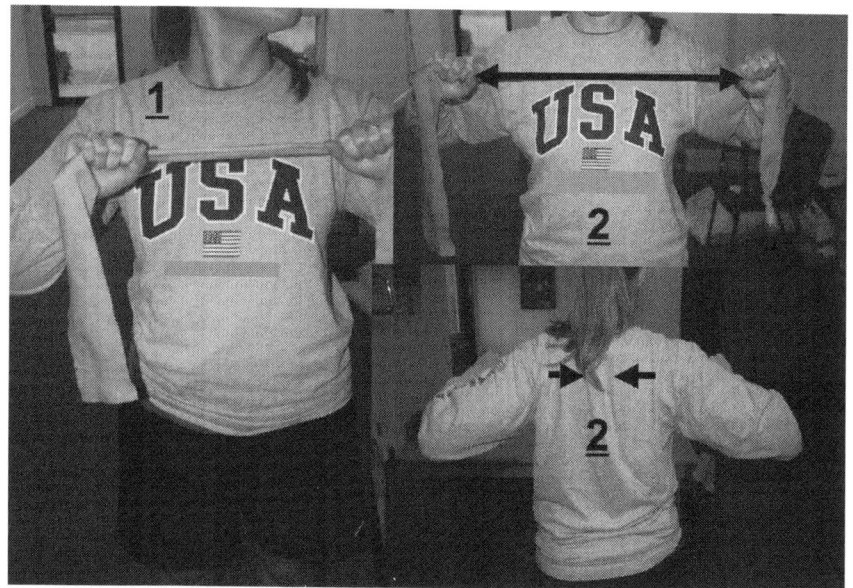

How to: The main purpose of this exercise is to squeeze your shoulder blades together. Start by holding the band with your hands close together and slowly pinch your shoulder blades together. If your hands separate any more than pictured in the top right, you are using your shoulders too much and your shoulder blades not enough.

## Serratus Punches

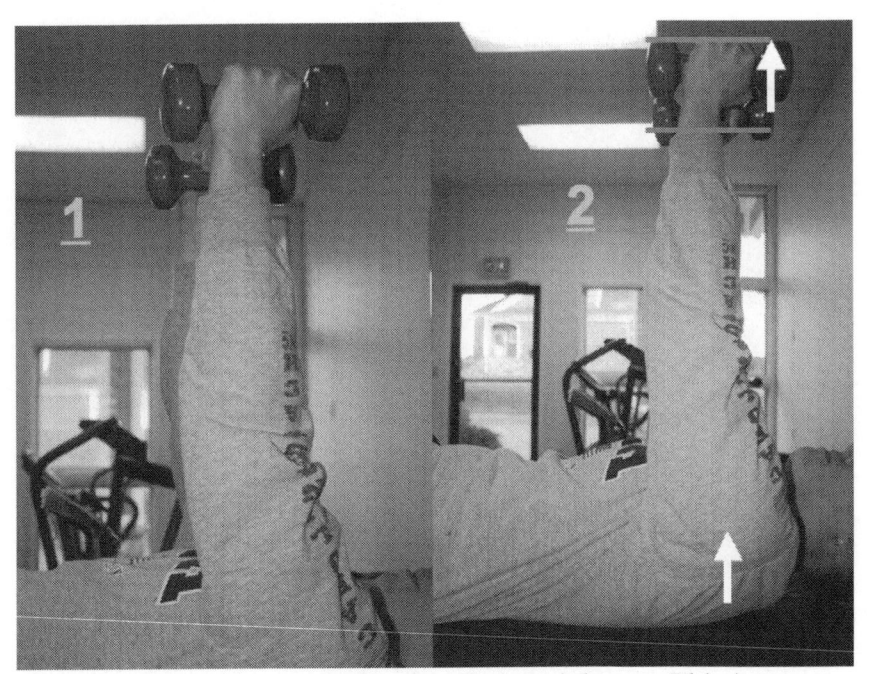

How to: Start with your arms extended straight up. This is a very small motion where you just reach your shoulders towards the ceiling. You are trying to strengthen your serratus anterior (punchers muscle).

## Shoulder Abduction

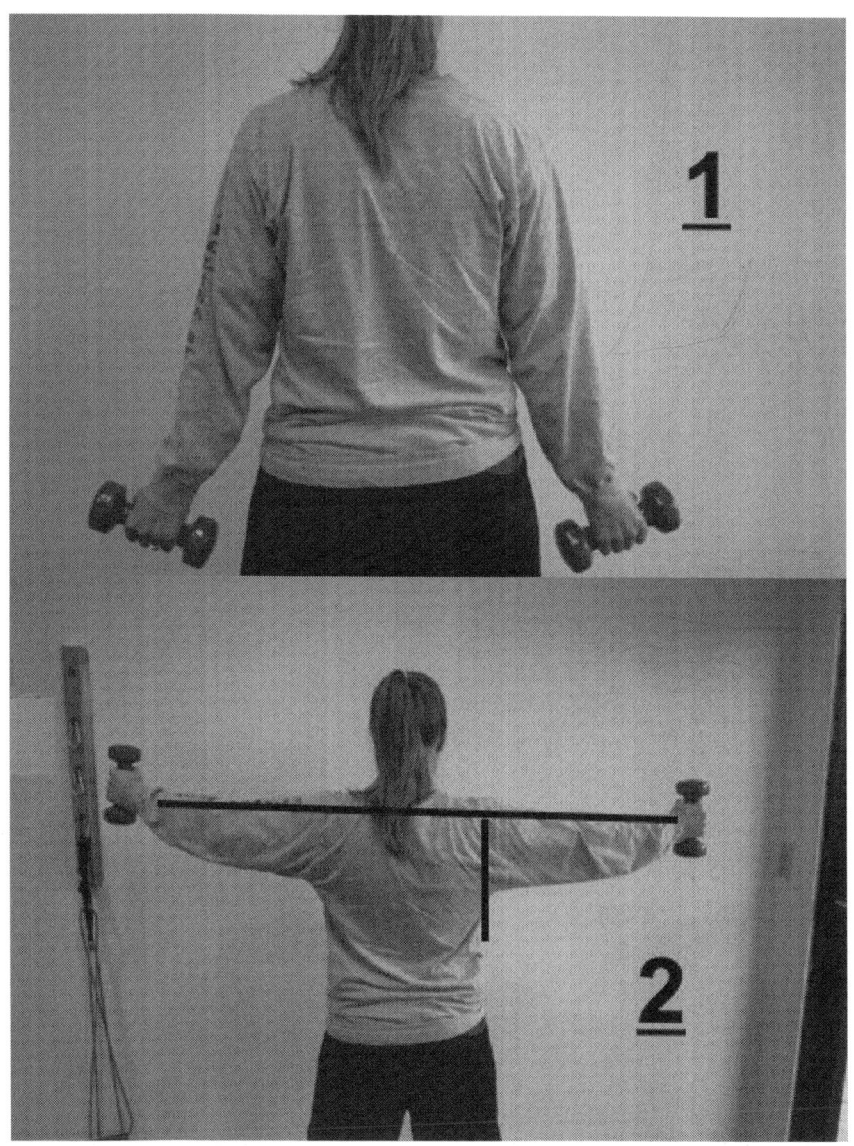

How to: Start with your elbows extended and resting at your side with your palms facing forward. Bring your arms up to shoulder level in line with the rest of your trunk. Hold for a brief second and slowly lower your arms back to the starting position.

## Shoulder External Rotation

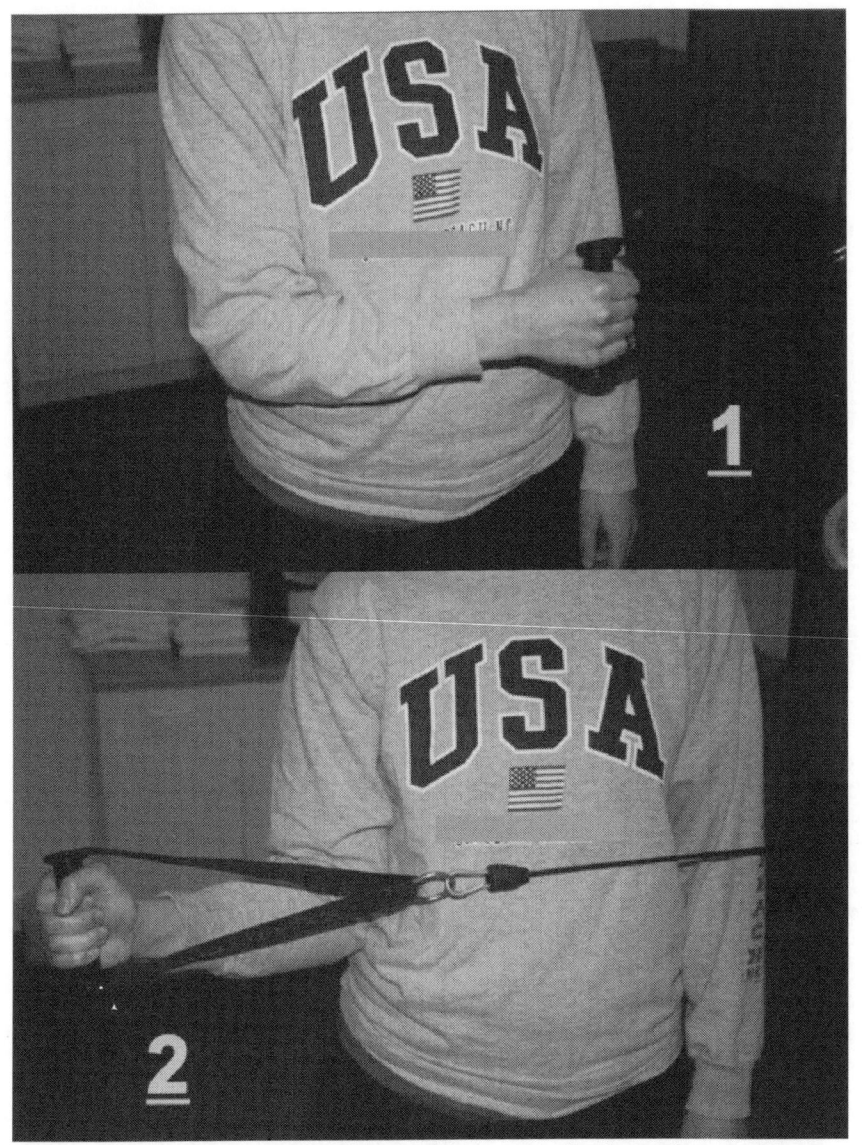

How to: Start with your elbow against your body and your elbow bent to 90°. Slowly rotate your arm out as far as you can keeping your elbow touching your side at all times. If it comes off your body, the weight is too heavy or you are rotating your arm too much.

## Shoulder Internal Rotation

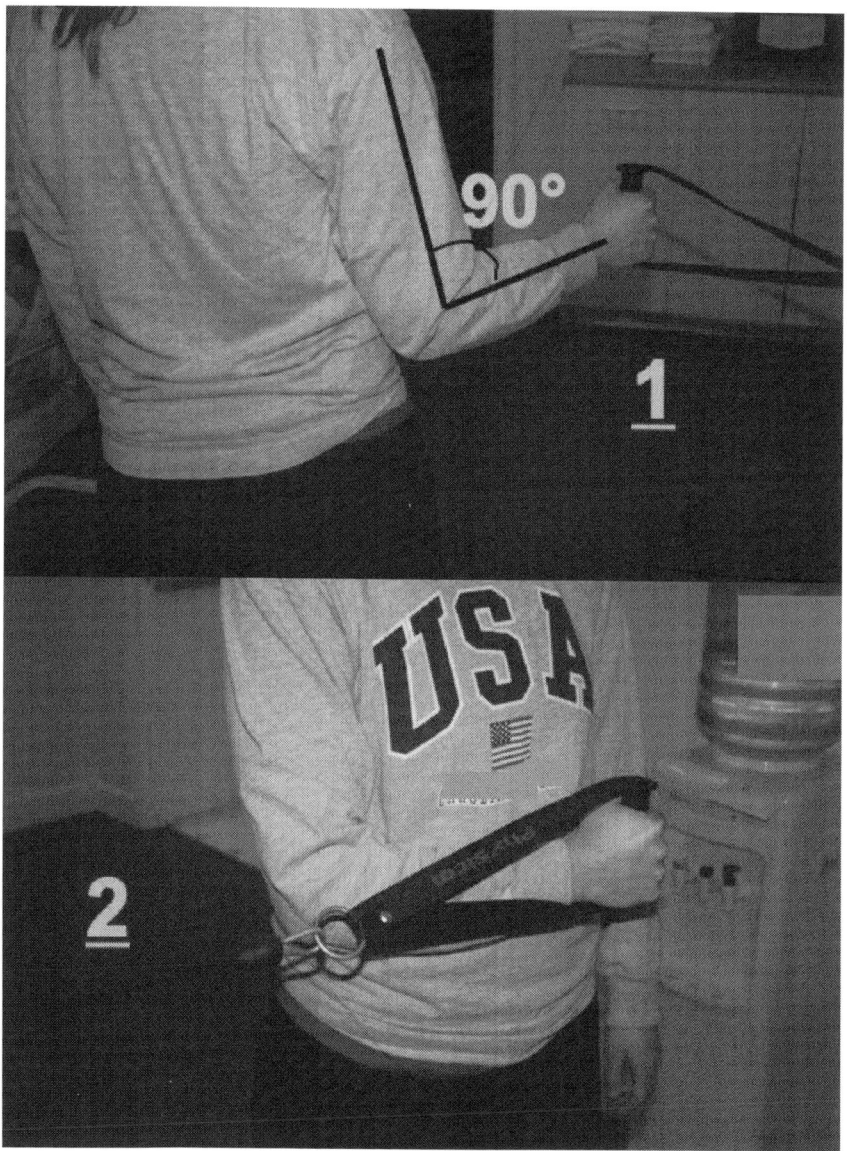

How to: Start with your elbow against your body and your elbow bent to 90°. Slowly rotate your arm in as far as you can keeping your elbow touching your side at all times. If it comes off your body, the weight is too heavy or you are rotating your arm too much.

## Side lying Hip Abduction

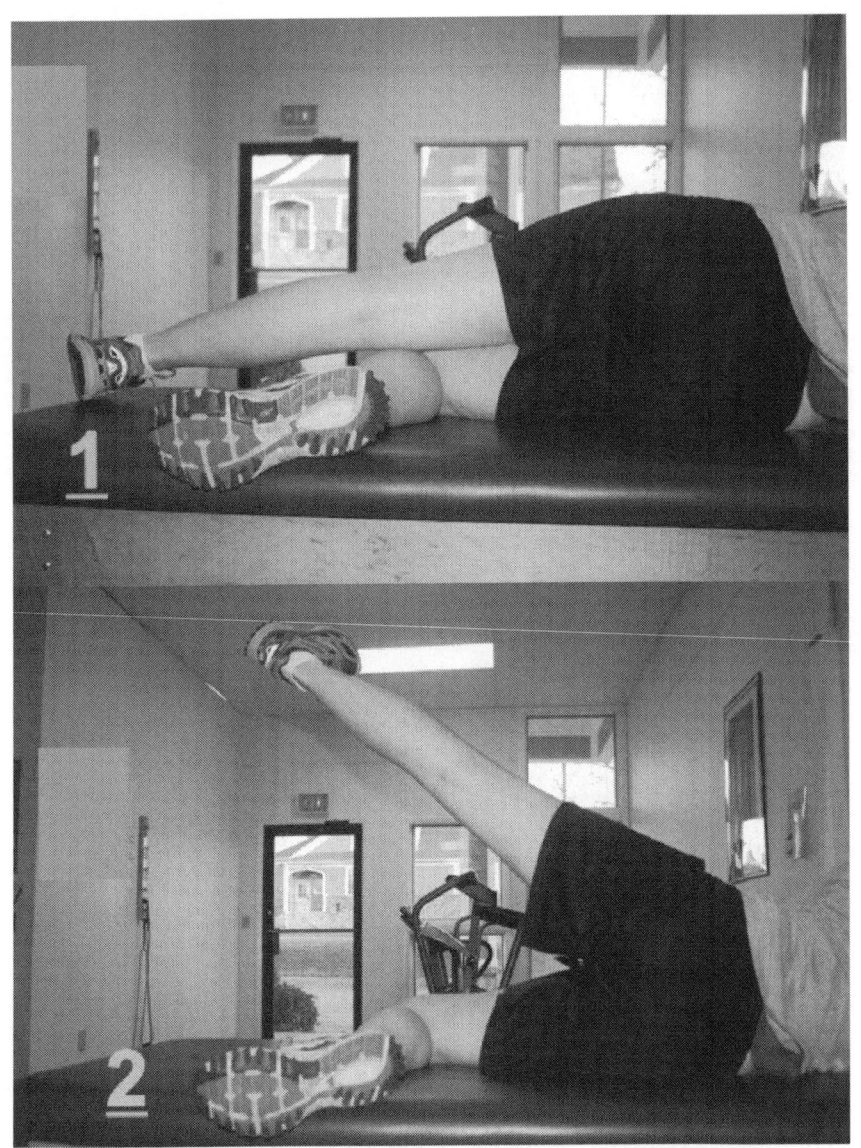

How to: Start on your side with the bottom leg bent for balance and the top leg straight. Next, lift the straight leg up towards the ceiling. Your leg should make a straight line from your heel to the top of your head. People commonly roll their hips back or bring their leg forward to make it easier. This will exercise a different muscle group. You should feel the strain on the side of your hip, not the front.

## Squats

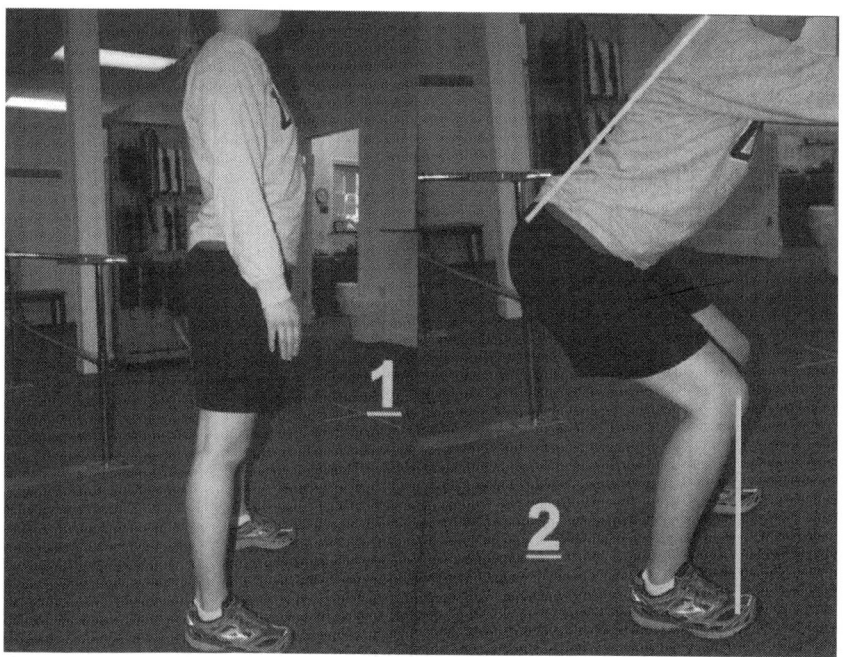

How to: Start with your legs straight and feet shoulder width apart. Slowly lower your backside as if you were sitting in a chair bending at the hips to maintain balance. Bend your knees without your knees coming past your toes (as shown above).

Step-Ups

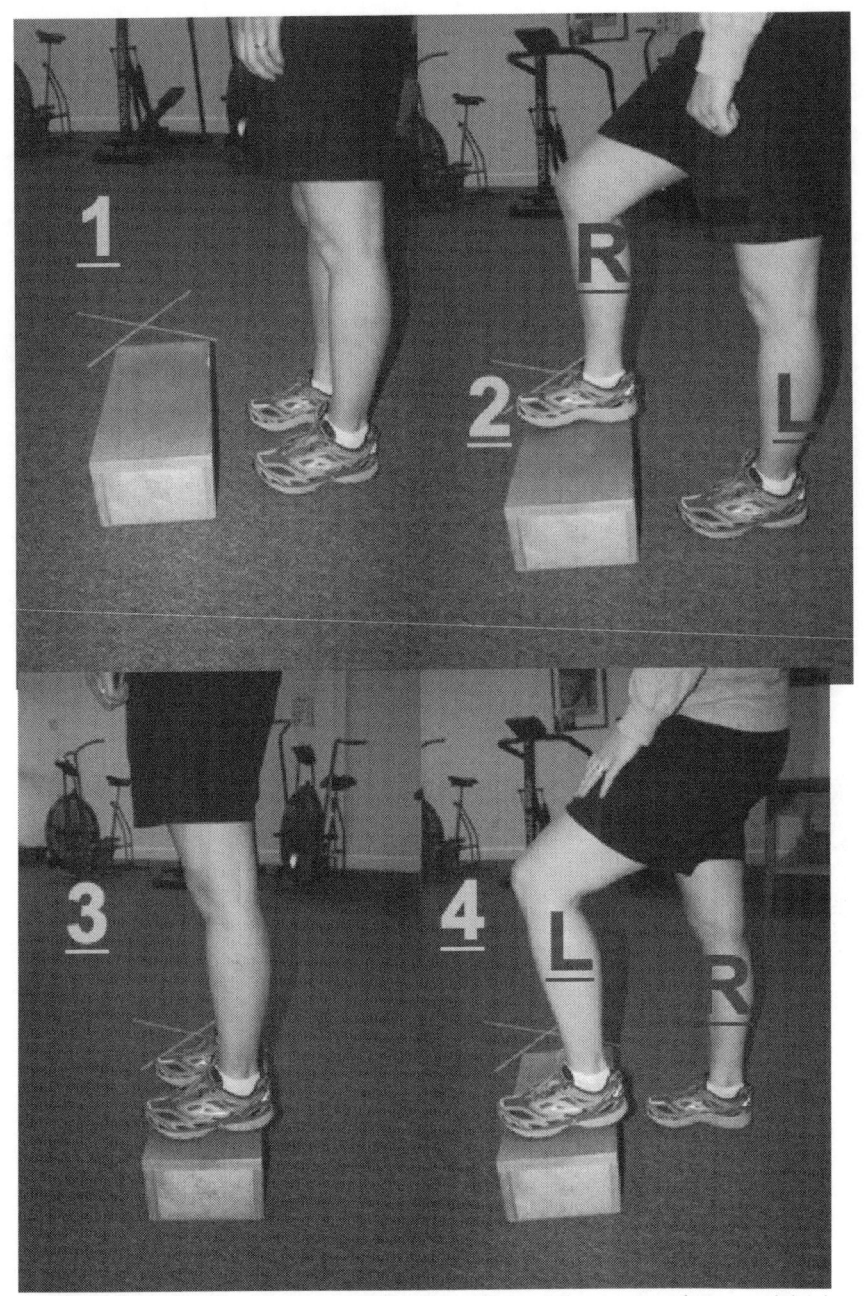

How to: Step up with the right, then left. Then step down with the right, then left. Repeat multiple times, then do repetitions with the left foot leading.

## Triceps Pushes

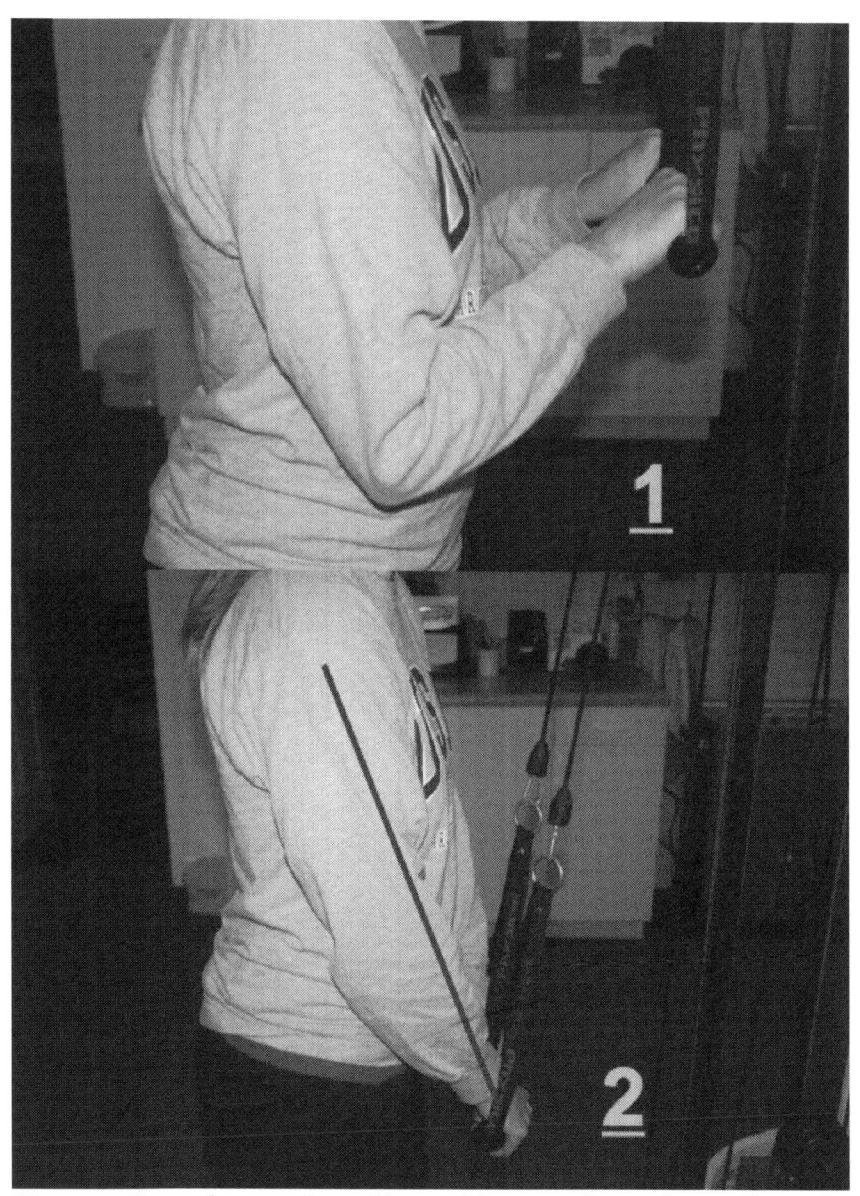

How to: Start close to the pulleys with your elbows bent. Extend your elbows and push straight down. All of the motion should be coming from your elbows and no motion from your shoulders.

## VOCABULARY

**Concentric contraction**: shortening the muscle against resistance. It would be the phase of a biceps curl where you are pulling the weight up. The phase where you lower it is considered eccentric (muscle lengthening against resistance).
**Cardiopulmonary System**: consists of your heart and lungs. It is responsible with getting rid of waste products (mainly $CO_2$), replenishing blood with oxygen, and pumping the blood out to the wanting tissue.
**Cardiovascular System**: consists of all the heart and vessels in the body. It is responsible for transporting blood all over the body.
**Eccentrics (Negatives):** a weightlifting technique where you add resistance as the muscle is lengthening. An example would be lowering a biceps curl very slowly back down to your side. The phase where you lift the biceps curl up is considered a concentric contraction because the muscle is shortening.
**$VO_2Max$**: in short, the maximum volume of $O_2$ your body can consume and use.

## **Before and After**

I thought it was only fair that I included a picture of me before and after I completed my own program. I lost a 30 pounds and have never felt better!

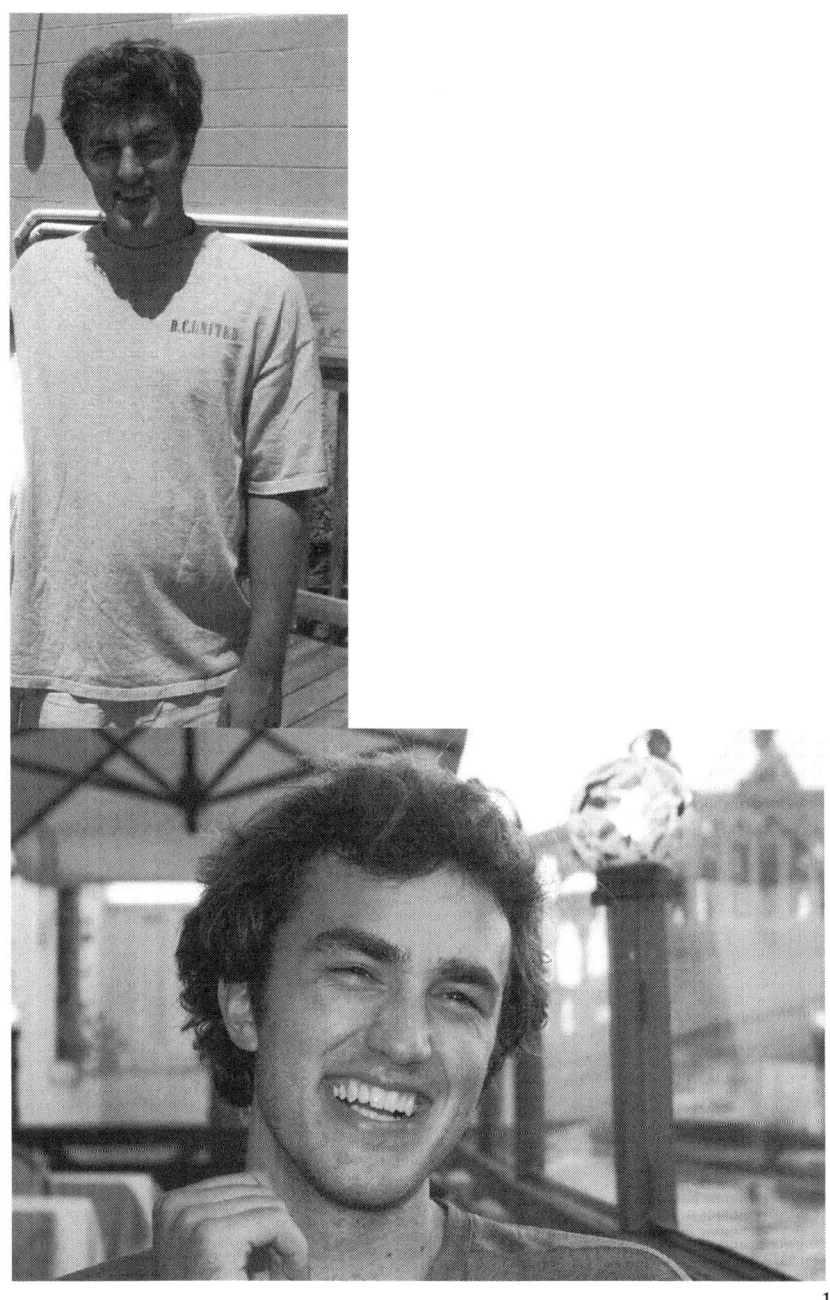

# Zazzle.com/SmartLife

Check out all the great Smart Life products!

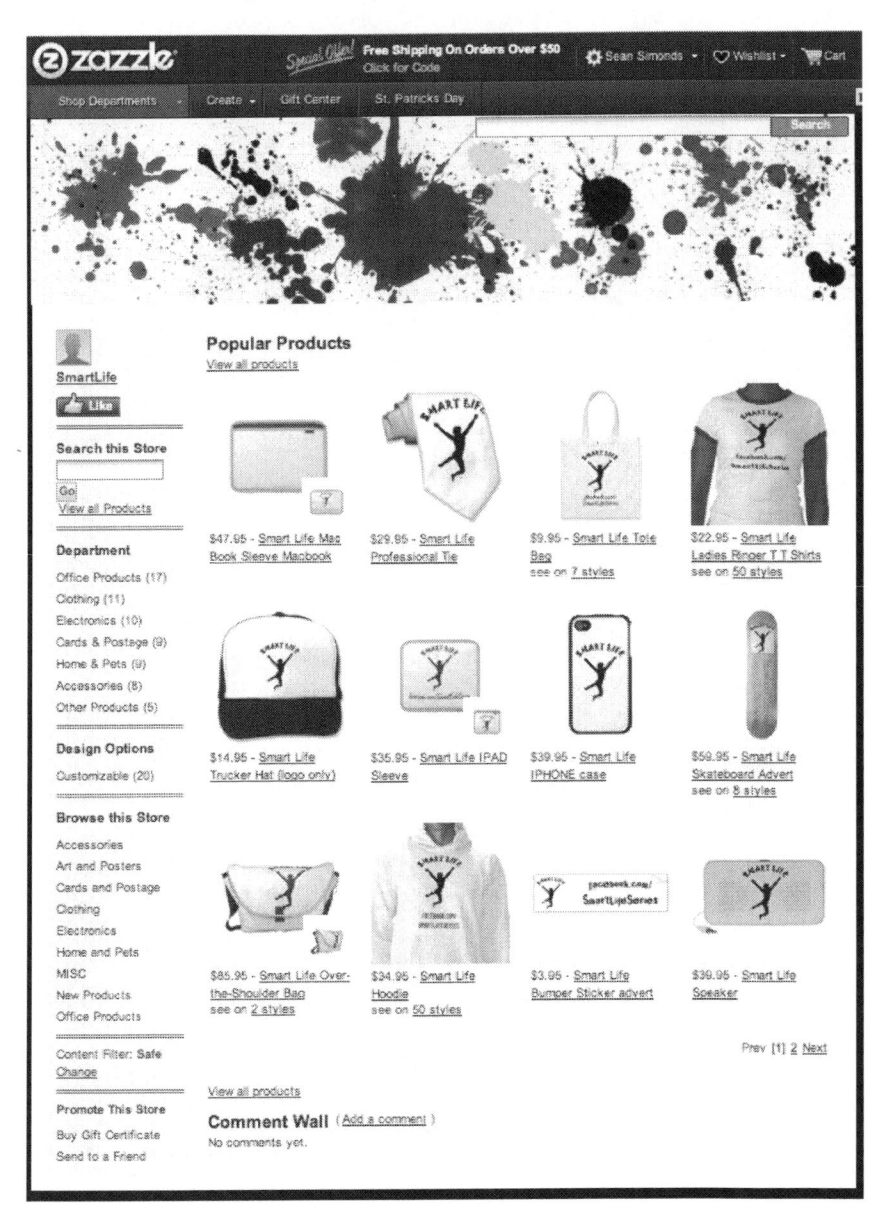

**http://smartlife-learninghealth.blogspot.com/**
Check the blog for extra information, videos, etc.!

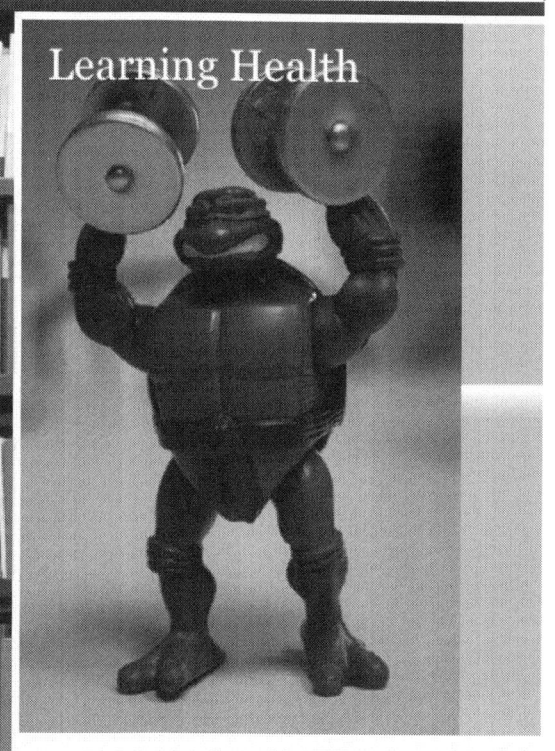

SUNDAY, MARCH 11, 2012

## Pulley Rows with Suspension Bands

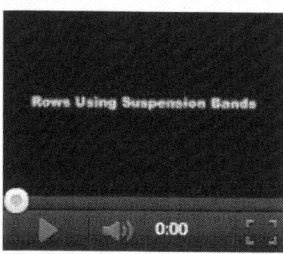

This is the first video in a hopefully long line of exercise videos. It is my hope that these videos give you guidance in how to properly perform certain exercises. I hope to include a variety of activities so that I can help a wide range of people. At the very least, maybe these videos will give you some new ideas to incorporate into your existing programs.

This video is showing you how to properly perform pulley rows using suspension bands. I have included a couple simple variations to help change it up.

Remember to keep your back/neck straight at all times, keep your feet planted, and start more perpendicular to the ground and move to a more parallel position as these get easier and easier.

As always, please send me any suggestions or questions you may have. My work email associated with the Smart Life Series is:

# Facebook.com/SmartLifeSeries
Come and check out all the new information and updates!

# **References**

1. Mayo Clinic Online at www.Mayoclinic.com
2. American Heart Association at www.heart.org
3. Smart Life/Learning Health Blog at http://smartlife-learninghealth.blogspot.com/
4. USDA at www.usda.gov
5. Magee, David. Orthopedic Physical Assessment. Saunders. 5th Ed. 2007
6. Dutton, Mark. Orthopedic Examination, Evaluation, and Intervention. McGraw Hill Medical. 2nd Ed. 2008
7. Goodman, C. Pathology: Implications for the Physical Therapist. Suanders. 3rd Ed. 2006
8. O'sullivan, S. Physical Rehabilitation. F.A. Davis Company. 5th Ed. 2006

Made in the USA
Charleston, SC
21 April 2012